Low

A Complete Guide to a Healthy Lifestyle Using
Real Foods and Real Science, How it Works,
How to Start, & More!

Dr. Michelle Ellen Gleen

directions contained herein is sole and complete. Under no conditions will the publisher be held liable for any reparation, damages, or monetary loss incurred as a result of the information contained herein, either explicitly or implicitly.

All copyrights not held by the publisher are owned by the respective author(s).

The information contained herein is provided solely for informational purposes and is therefore universal. The information is presented without contract or assurance of any kind.

The trademarks are used without the trademark owner's consent, and the trademark is published without the trademark owner's permission or support. All trademarks and brands mentioned in this book are solely for clarity purposes and are owned by their respective owners, who are not affiliated with this document.

Free Bonus

Download my **"Keto Cookbook with 60+ Keto Recipes For Your Personal Enjoyment"** Ebook For **FREE!**

The **Keto Diet Cookbook** is a collection of **60+ delicious recipes** that are easy and fun to make in the comfort of your own home. It gives you the exact *recipes that you can use to prepare meals for any moment of the day, breakfast, lunch, dinner, and even dessert.*

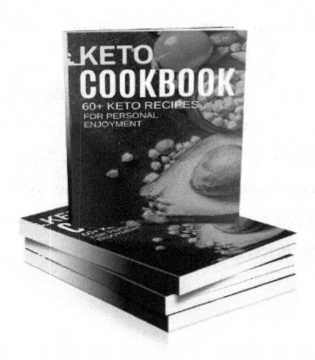

You don't need 5 different cookbooks with a ton of recipes to live a healthy and fun lifestyle. *You just need a*

good and efficient one and that is what the **Keto Diet Cookbook** is.

Click the URL below to Download the Book For FREE, and also Subscribe for Free books, giveaways, and new releases by me. https://mayobook.com/drmichelle

Other Books

1. Low Carb Diet: 100 Essential Flavorful Recipes For Quick & Easy Low-Carb Homemade Cooking
2. Low Carb Diet: A Complete Guide to a Healthy Lifestyle Using Real Foods and Real Science, How it Works, How to Start, & More!
3. Alkaline Diet: The Secret to Healthy Living with Alkaline Foods (Healthy Food Lifestyle)
4. Brain Cancer Awareness: How to Help Your Brain Fight Brain Cancer
5. Trigger Points: The New Self Treatment Guide to Pain Relief
6. Skin Tag Removal: How To Get Rid of Your Skin Tags in Simple Steps
7. Apple Cider Vinegar: A Quick, Easy, and Affordable Guide to the Health Benefits, and Healing Power of Apple Cider Vinegar (ACV)
8. Apple Cider Vinegar: The Amazing Guide on The Uses of ACV For Numerous Health Conditions, and How to Make it from Home
9. Dr. Sebi Cookbook: Alkaline Diet Nutritional Guide with Sea moss, Medicinal Herbal Teas, Smoothies, Desserts, Mushroom, Salads, Soups & More, to ... with 100+ Recipes

10. The Alkaline Diet Cookbook: Your Guide to Eating More Alkaline Foods, and Less Acidic Foods For Healthy Living (Healthy Food Lifestyle)

11. Ketogenic Diet For Beginners: Your Complete Keto Guide and Cookbook with Low Carb, High-Fat Recipes For Living The Keto Lifestyle

12. Anti Inflammatory Diet Cookbook For Beginners: 3-Week Quick & Delicious Meal Plan with Easy Recipes to Heal The Immune Systems and Restore Overall Health

Table of Contents

LOW CARB DIET 1

FREE BONUS 4

OTHER BOOKS 6

INTRODUCTION 15

CHAPTER 1 23

    Low-Carbohydrate Diet... 23

    Definition and classification 24

        Macronutrient ratios 24

        Foodstuffs 25

    Adoption and Advocacy 26

    Carbohydrate-Insulin Hypothesis 27

    Health Aspects 29

        Adherence 29

        Body Weight 29

        Cardiovascular Health 30

        Diabetes 31

    Exercise and Fatigue 34

    Ketogenic Diet 34

    Safety 35

    History 37

        First Descriptions 37

        Modern low-carbohydrate diets 38

CHAPTER 2 40

    Popular Methods to Execute a Low Carb Diet 40

An Average Low Carb Diet...40

Ketogenic Diet...42

Low-Carb, High-Fat (LCHF)...44

Low Carb Paleo Diet...44

The Atkins Diet..45

Eco-Atkins...46

Zero-Carb..47

Low carb Mediterranean Diet...48

DOES IT AID WEIGHT LOSS?...49

PURPOSE...50

DIET DETAILS...50

CHAPTER 3 53

TYPICAL FOODS FOR A LOW CARB DIET...53

RESULTS..54

Weight Loss...54

Other Health Advantages...54

RISKS..56

A LOW CARB MEAL PLAN AND MENU TO BOOST YOUR HEALTH..............57

Foods to avoid...58

Foods to Eat..59

Foods You Can Eat..60

LOW CARB MENU FOR A WEEK...61

HEALTHY, LOW CARB SNACKS..64

A SIMPLE LOW CARB GROCERY LIST..65

CHAPTER 4 68

BEST LOW CARB VEGETABLES..68

Bell Peppers..68

Broccoli...69

Asparagus...70

Mushrooms 70

Zucchini 71

Spinach 72

Avocados 73

Cauliflower 74

Green Beans 75

Lettuce 75

Garlic 76

Kale 77

Cucumbers 78

Brussels Sprouts 78

Celery 79

Tomatoes 80

Radishes 81

Onions 81

Eggplant 82

Cabbage 83

Artichokes 84

CHAPTER 5 85

Myths About Low Carb Diets 85

They're just a fad 85

Hard to stick with 86

A lot of the weight loss comes from water 87

Harmful to the heart 88

They work because people eat fewer calories 90

They lessen your consumption of healthy plant foods 91

Ketosis is a dangerous metabolic state 91

The human brain needs carbs to operate 93

They destroy physical performance 94

Common Low carb Mistakes (and how to avoid them) 95

Eating Too Many Carbs 96

Eating too much Protein 96

The fear of eating fat 97

Not Replenishing Sodium 98

Quitting Too Early 99

C H A P T E R   6 .... **102**

WAYS TO REDUCE YOUR CARBOHYDRATE INTAKE 102

Eliminate Sugar-Sweetened Drinks 102

Cut back on Bread 103

Stop Drinking Juice 104

Choose Low carb Snacks 104

Eat Eggs or Additional Low carb Breakfast Foods 106

Use These Sweeteners instead of Sugar 107

Ask for Veggies instead of Potatoes or Breads at Restaurants 108

Substitute Low carb Flours for Wheat Flour 109

Replace Milk with Almond or Coconut Milk 110

Emphasize Non-Starchy Veggies 111

Choose Dairy That's Low in Carbs 112

Eat Healthy High-Protein Foods 113

Prepare Foods with Healthy Fats 114

Reading Food Labels 115

Count Carbs Having a Nutrition Tracker 116

C H A P T E R   7 .... **118**

JUNK FOODS YOU CAN EAT ON THE LOW CARB DIET 118

Sub in a tub 118

KFC Grilled Chicken 119

Tea or coffee with cream 120

Chipotle salad or bowl 121

Lettuce-wrapped burger 122

Panera Breads power breakfast bowl 123

Buffalo wings 124

Bacon or Sause and Eggs 125

Arby's sandwich with no bun or bread 126

Antipasto salad 127

Subway double chicken chopped salad 128

Burrito bowl 129

McDonald's breakfast sandwich with no bread 130

Arby's roast turkey farmhouse salad 130

C H A P T E R   8 132

FOODS TO AVOID (OR LIMIT) ON THE LOW CARB DIET 132

Bread and grains 132

Some fruit 134

Starchy vegetables 135

Pasta 136

Cereal 137

Beer 138

Sweetened Yogurt 139

Juice 139

Low-fat and fat-free salad dressings 140

Beans and Legumes 141

Honey or Sugar in any form 142

Chips and Crackers 144

Milk 144

Gluten-free Cooked Food 145

C H A P T E R   9 147

REASONS YOU ARE NOT LOSING WEIGHT ON THE LOW CARB DIET 147

You Are Losing Weight, You Just Don't Understand It 147

You're not reducing on Carbohydrates Enough 148

You're Stressed Regularly *149*

You're Not Consuming Real Food *150*

You're Eating Too Many Nuts *151*

You are not Sleeping Enough *152*

You're eating too much Dairy *153*

You're Not Exercising Right (or whatsoever) *154*

You're Eating Too Many "Healthy" Sugars *155*

You Might Have a Health Condition Making Things Difficult *156*

You're Constantly Eating *157*

You're Cheating too often *158*

You're Ingesting too many Calories *159*

You do not have Realistic Expectations *159*

You've Been "Cutting" for too much time *160*

C H A P T E R   1 0 .... **162**

HOW MUCH CARBS SHOULD YOU EAT PER DAY TO LOSE EXCESS WEIGHT? 162

WHY WOULD YOU EAT FEWER CARBS? 162

CARBS INTAKE 164

HOW TO DECIDE YOUR DAILY CARB INTAKE 165

Consuming 100-150 Grams each day *166*

Ingesting 50-100 grams each day *166*

Consuming less than 50 grams each day *167*

IT'S VITAL THAT YOU EXPERIMENT 167

LOW CARB JUNK FOOD THAT ARE UNHEALTHY. 168

LOW CARBOHYDRATE DIETS ASSIST YOU TO BURN FAT 169

FRUITS AND LOW-CARB 172

PASS YOUR CARB BUDGET WISELY 174

HOW ABOUT FRUCTOSE? 175

FRUIT IS HEALTHY 176

LOW CARB FRUITS 177

C H A P T E R   1 1 .... **179**

Low Carb Kitchen Gadgets 179

    Silicone Bakeware 179

    Kitchen Scales 179

    Measuring Cups and Measuring Spoons 180

    Spiralizer 180

    Non-stick Frying Pan 181

    Stick Blender 181

    Glass Storage Containers 181

    Food Processor 182

    Figure Out How to Enjoy Your Slow Cooker 182

    Baking Mat 182

    Power Blender 183

Ways To Stay Low on Carbohydrate When You Don't Want to Cook 183

    Drink coffee or tea 184

    Eat low carb snacks 184

    Reheat leftovers 185

    Do minimal cooking 185

    Fast intermittently 186

NOTE 187

FREE BONUS 188

FEEDBACK 190

ABOUT THE AUTHOR 192

OTHER BOOKS 194

Introduction

Our food has nutrient, and the three primary nutrients are carbohydrates, proteins, and fats. We might decide to favor or restrict these macronutrients that allow us to classify diets as high-carb, low-fat, high-protein, or low-carb. Whenever we restrict carbs to below 130g each day, we are taking a diet plan that is lower in carbohydrates. What happens when we are on a low carb diet?

And how low on carb can we go?

When you eat fewer carbs, you get the remaining calories that your body needs to help to make fuel from your other two sources: fat and protein. Thus, a low carb diet is a diet saturated in protein and healthy fats. Why do people choose to eat more body fat and reduce carbs? Isn't that against good sense?

Good, no.

Fats will always be blamed for obesity, perhaps because obesity means being fat.

Based on that belief, low-fat foods had been invented to reduce obesity and make people slim. The truth is, the so-called low-fat foods had been the start of the obesity epidemics because, while these were deprived of most

15

fats, those foods were filled with all of the bad carbs. Being that they are less calorie-rich, it is possible to eat more carbs than the body needs. So, what happened to the excess carbs? Your body turned them into fat.

People choose low carb diets because they would like to shed weight. So how does it work? Sugar and starches, i.e., carbohydrates, make our blood sugar oscillate and have a tendency to heighten insulin (fat-storing hormone) levels. Sooner or later, your body can't produce enough insulin to normalize blood sugar, i.e., you have Type 2 diabetes. Consequently, if we remove starches and sugar from our diet, we get stabilized blood sugar and reduced insulin levels.

You become healthy, avoid obesity and be in perfect shape. Once you don't feed your body on fat, it begins to feed on fat and protein.

Plus, your body will never feel like it requires to eat just as much since sugar levels are stabilized and they don't fall and rise triggering hunger regularly.

Facts about Carbohydrates

Carbs are the most abundant type of bio-molecules, and they're mainly in charge of transporting energy.

Carbohydrates are informally known as carbs and so are starches or sugars. Carbs are an important food source.

However, they turn into a problem whenever we give the body too many carbohydrates. Actually, we give the body a lot of that it can't store them as glycogen and must turn them into fat. Too many carbs make us fat.

You'd be challenged to get any dietitian, doctor, or doctor anywhere who agrees that the normal United States diet is ideal.

As a population, we tend to eat a lot of junk, mostly out of convenience but also just out of habit. We've become familiar with a whole lot of foods that unfortunately have some negative impacts on our health and wellness, especially when consumed excessively. What a lot of people don't understand is that; a nutritious diet means what makes up a meal and not exactly how much we eat. Simply reducing food portion sizes isn't likely to cut it.

That's where the reduced carb diet comes in. Going low on carbohydrates is not about eliminating bread from your diet, but understanding very clearly where all carbs come from in our diet, and ensuring we are managing our carb intake along with maintaining a healthy lifestyle including exercise along with other habits for general well-being.

Why the Low Carb Lifestyle?

The amount of carbs in the United States diet is greater than what's nutritionally required, plus the impacts of the diet have already established some drastic impacts on the overall health of people.

Excessive carbohydrate intake continues to be linked with excess weight, but carbs also affect blood sugar levels and insulin amounts, cholesterol, crystals levels, blood pressure, and more. Some people experience more significant effects than others; however, the implications aren't something anyone should ignore.

Now, this isn't to say we have to possess a knee-jerk reaction or imply that carbs are bad. Some carbs are necessary to maintain a sound body, and a balanced diet will need some carbohydrates in it. However, the main element is understanding how much carbs are in the meals we eat, and the type of carbs they may be. This way, we can develop a better diet plan and begin to create healthier food choices so our bodies are getting just what is needed, rather than loading up an excessive amount of one thing or another.

Types of Carbs

There are three main types of carbohydrates that people have to be aware of. Each has different characteristics, so when you get down the road to a minimal-carb life, you'll learn how to manage each one through wise food choices and carb counting techniques. Listed below are the three types of carbs:

Sugars - Also called simple carbohydrates, sugars are located in an extremely wide selection of foods. Sugars can either be natural, like the sugars you'll find in fruits or dairy, or processed sugars that have been put into foods during production. Simple sugars are often broken down and digested by your body.

Starches - Another common name for starches is complex carbohydrates, and they are found mostly in grains like wheat and wheat products, vegetables like potatoes, and various types of beans. Complex carbohydrates are converted during digestion into simple carbohydrates (sugars); therefore, they are typically absorbed more slowly into the body.

Fibers - Although necessary to having a healthy digestive system, most of the fiber we intake is indigestible by the body. Nevertheless, it is a critical part of your digestive health, keeps your body regular, and in addition, helps to keep your stomach full when you've eaten.

It's very important for beginners on the reduced carb diet to start by paying attention to nourishment labels on the foods they eat and being attentive to the quantity of these three carbohydrates.

The number of carbs you'll find in a few common products may surprise you, as there tend to be more than you'd expect. For instance, a lot of people would agree that fresh mangoes or some ripe cherries are a wonderful healthy snack; however, they are fruits that contain a number of the highest matters of sugar, therefore should be ingested on a minimal carb diet only in careful moderation.

Different low Carbohydrate Diets

While we won't go into the detailed specifics of every type of diet program here, and you should always check with your doctor before starting any new diet program, there are many popular low carbohydrate diets that you might consider in case you feel that this could be right for you.

Below are a few of the normal plans that low carbohydrate dieters are following:

The Atkins Diet - You've probably heard about that one. The common low carbohydrate diet, the Atkins Diet targets restricting carb intake and transitioning the body's metabolism to burn up excess fat rather than glucose.

The Dukan Diet - The dietary plan requires a slightly different approach and advises a far more moderate method of carb restrictions as well as the moderation of fat intake. The dietary plan has four phases to gradually adjust carb intake.

Dr. Poon's Metabolic Diet - Concentrating on a low carbohydrate, low sodium, and moderate fat intake, the dietary plan was made to achieve weight loss to ease the consequences of medical ailments such as diabetes, hypertension, and raised cholesterol.

The G.We Diet - Also called the *Glycemic Index Diet*, the dietary plan categorizes carbs by how promptly these are digested by your body and how quickly they increase blood sugar. It recommends which foods to reduce, or cut out entirely to accomplish weight loss.

Success in the Low Carb Diet

Many people have achieved their health goals through a minimal carb diet. Whether for weight loss, easing the consequences of diabetes, or combating high blood pressure, you will find inspirational stories from around the world that display the difference in a minimal carb lifestyle could make.

If you believe the low carb diet may be right for you personally, speak to your doctor and start taking actions to a healthy and happier future.

Chapter 1

Low-Carbohydrate Diet

A low-carbohydrate diet restricts the quantity of carbohydrate-rich foods - such as bread - in the dietary plan.

Low-carbohydrate diets restrict carbohydrate consumption under the common diet. Foods saturated in carbohydrates (e.g., sugar, bread, pasta) are reduced and replaced with foods containing an increased percentage of fat and protein (e.g., meat, chicken, fish, shellfish, eggs, cheese, nuts, and seeds), as well as low carb foods (e.g., spinach, kale, chard, collards, along with other fibrous vegetables).

There's an insufficient standardization of just how much of low-carbohydrate diets will need to have, which has complicated research. One definition, from the American Academy of Family Doctors, specifies low-carbohydrate diets is having significantly less than 20% carbohydrate content.

There are absolutely no good evidence that low-carbohydrate dieting gives any particular health advantages apart from weight loss, where low-carbohydrate diets achieve outcomes much like other diets, as weight loss is mainly dependent on calorie restriction and adherence.

An extreme type of low-carbohydrate diet - *the ketogenic diet* - is made like a medical diet for treating epilepsy. Through celebrity endorsement, it has turned into a popular weight-loss crash diet, but there is absolutely no proof of any distinctive benefit for this function, and it could have several initial side effects.

Definition and classification

Macronutrient ratios

The macronutrient ratios of low-carbohydrate diets aren't standardized.

By 2018 the conflicting definitions of "low-carbohydrate" diets have complicated research on this subject.

The American Academy of Family Doctors defines low-carbohydrate diets as diets that restrict carbohydrate intake to 20 to 60 grams (g) each day, typically significantly less than 20% of calorie consumption. A

2016 overview of low-carbohydrate diets classified diets with 50g of carbohydrate each day (significantly less than 10% of total calories) as "Surprisingly low" and diets with 40% of calories from carbohydrates as "mild" low-carbohydrate diets. The United Kingdom National Health Service advises that *"carbohydrates should be the body's main way to obtain energy in a healthy, balanced diet."*

Foodstuffs

Like additional vegetables, curly kale is a food that's low in carbohydrates.

There is evidence that the product quality, as opposed to the quantity, of carbohydrates in a diet, is very important to health, high-fiber slow-digesting carbohydrate-rich foods are healthy while highly-refined and sugary foods are less so. People choosing a diet for health issues must have their diet tailored to their specific requirements. For those who have metabolic conditions, a diet plan with approximately 40-50% carbohydrate is preferred.

Most vegetables are low- or moderate-carbohydrate foods (in a few low-carbohydrate diets, fiber is excluded since it isn't a nutritive carbohydrate). Some vegetables, such as potatoes, carrots, maize (corn), and rice are saturated in starch. Most low-carbohydrate weight loss plans accommodate vegetables such as *broccoli, spinach, kale, lettuce, cucumbers, cauliflower, peppers & most green-leafy vegetables.*

Adoption and Advocacy

The National Academy of Medicine recommends a regular average of 130 g of carbohydrates each day. The FAO and WHO similarly advise that all dietary energy results from carbohydrates. Low-carbohydrate diets aren't a choice recommended in the 2015-2020 edition of Dietary Guidelines for Americans, which instead recommends a minimal fat diet.

Carbohydrate continues to be wrongly accused to be a uniquely "fattening" macronutrient, misleading many dieters into compromising the nutritiousness of the diet through the elimination of carbohydrate-rich food. Low-carbohydrate diet proponents emphasize research saying that low-carbohydrate diets can initially cause slightly greater fat loss when compared to a balanced diet, but such an advantage will not persist. In the long-term successful weight, maintenance depends on calorie consumption, rather than on macronutrient ratios.

The public is becoming confused incidentally where some diets, like the Zone diet as well as the South Beach diet are promoted as "low-carbohydrate" when they can be properly called "medium" carbohydrate diets.

Carbohydrate-Insulin Hypothesis

Low-carbohydrate diet advocates including Gary Taubes and David Ludwig possess proposed a *"carbohydrate-insulin hypothesis"* where carbohydrates are reported to be uniquely fattening because they raise insulin levels and cause fat to build up unduly.

The hypothesis seems to run counter to known human biology whereby there is no proof of such association between your actions of insulin, fat accumulation, and obesity. The hypothesis predicted that low-carbohydrate dieting would provide a "metabolic advantage" of increased energy expenditure equal to 400-600 kcal (kilo calorie)/daily in accord with the promise from the Atkin's diet: a "high-calorie way to remain slim forever."

With funding from the Laura and John Arnold Foundation, in 2012, Taubes co-founded the Nourishment Science Initiative (NuSI), to raise over $200 million to attempt a "Manhattan Project for Nutrition" and validate the hypothesis. Intermediate results, published in the American Journal of Clinical Nutrition didn't provide convincing proof of any advantage to some low-carbohydrate diets when compared with diets of other composition - ultimately an extremely low-calorie, ketogenic diet (of 5% carbohydrate) "had not been connected with significant lack of fat mass" in comparison to a non-specialized diet using the same calories; there is no useful *"metabolic advantage."*

In 2017 Kevin Hall, an NIH (National Institutes of Health) researcher employed to assist with the project, wrote that this carbohydrate-insulin hypothesis has been falsified by experiment. Hall wrote, "the rise in obesity prevalence could be primarily because of increased consumption of processed carbohydrates, however, the mechanisms will tend to be quite not the same as those proposed from the carbohydrate-insulin model."

Health Aspects

Adherence

It's been repeatedly discovered that in the long-term, all diets using the same calorific value perform the same for weight loss, aside from the main one differentiating factor of how well people can faithfully follow the dietary plan. A report comparing groups taking low-fat, low-carbohydrate and Mediterranean diets for half a year in the low-carbohydrate diet still had a lot of people sticking with it, but thereafter the problem reversed: at 2 years the low-carbohydrate group had the best incidence of lapses and dropouts. This can be because of the comparatively limited food selection of low-carbohydrate diets.

Body Weight

Studies show that people slimming down having a low-carbohydrate diet, in comparison to a low-fat diet, have very slightly more excess weight loss initially, equal to approximately 100kcal/daily but that the benefit diminishes as time passes and it is ultimately insignificant. The Endocrine Society stated that "when calorie consumption is held constant, body-fat accumulation will not look like affected by actually very pronounced changes in the quantity of fat vs. carbohydrate in the dietary plan."

Most of the studies comparing low-fat vs. low-carbohydrate dieting have been of low quality and studies that reported large effects have garnered disproportionate attention compared to those that are methodologically sound.

A 2018 review said, "higher-quality meta-analyses reported little if any difference in weight loss between the two diets." Low-quality meta-analyses have tended to report favorably on the result of low-carbohydrate diets: a systematic review reported that 8 out of 10 meta-analyses assessed whether weight-loss outcomes might have been suffering from publication bias, and 7 of these concluded positively.

A 2017 review figured many diets, including low-carbohydrate diets, achieve similar weight loss outcomes, that are mainly dependent on calorie restriction and adherence as opposed to the kind of diet.

Cardiovascular Health

By 2016 it was unclear whether low-carbohydrate dieting had any beneficial influence on cardiovascular health, though such diets could cause high LDL cholesterol levels, which have a threat of atherosclerosis in the long run. Potential favorable changes in triglyceride and HDL cholesterol values should be weighed against potential unfavorable changes in LDL and total cholesterol values.

Some randomized control trials show that low-carbohydrate diets, especially very low-carbohydrate diets, perform much better than low-fat diets in improving cardio metabolic risk factors in the long run, suggesting that low-carbohydrate diets are a viable option alongside low-fat diets for people vulnerable to coronary disease.

There is poor-quality proof of the result of different diets on reducing or preventing high blood pressure, nonetheless, it suggests the low-carbohydrate diet is probably the better-performing one, as the DASH diet (Dietary Methods to Stop Hypertension) performs best.

Diabetes

There is little evidence for the potency of low-carbohydrate diets for those who have Type 1 diabetes. For several people, it might be feasible to check out a low-carbohydrate regime coupled with carefully-managed insulin dosing. This is hard to keep up and there are concerns about potential adverse health effects due to the dietary plan. Generally, people who have Type 1 diabetes should follow an individualized diet program.

The proportion of carbohydrates in a diet isn't from the threat of type 2 diabetes, although there is some evidence that diets containing certain high-carbohydrate items - such as sugar-sweetened drinks or white rice - are connected with an increased risk. Some evidence indicates that eating fewer carbohydrate foods may reduce biomarkers of Type 2 diabetes.

A 2018 report on Type 2 diabetes from the American Diabetes Association (ADA) and the European Association for the analysis of Diabetes (EASD) discovered that a low-carbohydrate diet may not be as effective as a Mediterranean diet for improving glycemic control, which although having a sound body weight is essential, "there is no single ratio of carbohydrate, proteins, and fat intake that's optimal for everyone with type 2 diabetes." There is no sound evidence that low-carbohydrate diets are better than a conventional nutritious diet, where carbohydrates take up more than 40% of calories consumed. Low-carbohydrate dieting does not have any influence on the kidney function of people who have type 2 diabetes.

Restricting carbohydrate consumption generally leads to improved glucose control, although without long-term fat loss. Low-carbohydrate diets can be handy to help people who have type 2 diabetes slim down, but "no approach has shown to become consistently superior."

Based on the ADA, people who have diabetes should be "developing healthy eating patterns instead of focusing on human being macronutrients, micronutrients, or single foods." They recommended the carbohydrates in a diet should come from "vegetables, legumes, fruits, dairy (milk and yogurt), and whole grains", while highly-refined foods and sweet drinks should be prevented. The ADA also wrote that "reducing carbohydrate intake for people with diabetes demonstrated the most evidence for improving glycemia and could be used in several eating patterns that meet individual needs and preferences."

For people with type 2 diabetes who can't meet up with the glycemic targets or where reducing anti-glycemic medications is important, the ADA says that low or very-low-carbohydrate diets are a viable approach.

Exercise and Fatigue

A low-carbohydrate diet is found to reduce the strength convenience of intense exercise, and depleted muscle glycogen after such actions is slowly replenished in case a low-carbohydrate diet is taken. Inadequate carbohydrate intake during athletic training causes metabolic acidosis, which might be responsible for poor performance.

Ketogenic Diet

The ketogenic diet is a high-fat, low-carbohydrate diet used to take care of drug-resistant childhood epilepsy.

In 2010, it became a crash diet for people trying to lose weight. Followers of the ketogenic diet might not achieve sustainable weight loss, as this involves strict carbohydrate abstinence, and maintaining the dietary plan is usually difficult. Possible risks of using the ketogenic diet in the future can has kidney stones, osteoporosis, or increased degrees of the crystals, a risk factor for gout.

Ketogenic diet (low carb diet) practice for weight loss has reportedly increased mortality rate (especially from cancer and heart problems), but mortality increase was just related to animal-based diets, whereas mortality was reduced with plant-based diets.

Safety

High and low-carbohydrate diets which are abundant with proteins and fats from animal-sourced foods might be connected with increased mortality. On the other hand, with plant-derived proteins and fats, there might be a decrease in mortality.

By 2018, research has paid little attention to the possible undesirable effects of carbohydrate-restricted dieting, particularly for micronutrient sufficiency, bone health insurance, and cancer risk. One poor meta-analysis reported that side effects could has *"constipation, headache, halitosis, muscle cramps, and general weakness."*

Ketosis induced with a low-carbohydrate diet has resulted in reported cases of ketoacidosis, a life-threatening condition. It has resulted in the suggestion that ketoacidosis is highly recommended as a potential hazard of low-carbohydrate dieting.

In a thorough systematic overview of 2018, Churuangsuk and colleagues reported that other case reports bring about concerns regarding other potential risks of low-carbohydrate dieting including hyperosmolar coma, Wernicke's encephalopathy, optic neuropathy from thiamine deficiency, acute coronary syndrome and panic.

Considerably restricting the proportion of carbohydrates in diet risks causing malnutrition, and may make it difficult to get enough soluble fiber to remain healthy.

By 2014 it appeared that with regards to the threat of death for those who have cardiovascular disease, the type of carbohydrates consumed is essential; diets relatively higher in fiber and whole grains result in a reduced threat of death from coronary disease in comparison to diets saturated in refined-grains.

History

First Descriptions

In 1797, John Rollo reported the results of treating two diabetic Army officers with a low-carbohydrate diet and medications. An extremely low-carbohydrate, ketogenic diet was the typical treatment for diabetes throughout the entire nineteenth century.

In 1863, William Banting, a formerly obese English undertaker and coffin maker, published "Letter on Corpulence Addressed to the general public," where he described an eating plan for weight control quitting loaf of bread, butter, milk, sugar, beer, and potatoes. His booklet was widely read; so much that some people used the word "Banting" for the experience now called "dieting."

In the first 1900s, Frederick Madison Allen developed an extremely restrictive short-term regime that was described by Walter R. Steiner in the 1916 annual convention with the Connecticut State Medical Society as The Starvation Treatment of Diabetes Mellitus. The dietary plan was often administered in a hospital to be able to better guarantee compliance and safety.

Modern low-carbohydrate diets

Additional low-carbohydrate diets in the 1960s had the environment Force diet along with the Drinking Man's Diet. In 1972, Robert Atkins published Dr. Atkins' Diet Revolution, which advocated the low-carbohydrate diet he previously successfully found in treating people in the 1960s. The book was a publishing success but was broadly criticized by the mainstream medical community to be dangerous and misleading, thereby limiting its appeal at that time.

The idea of the glycemic index originated in 1981 by David Jenkins to take into account variances in the speed of digestion of various kinds of carbohydrates. This idea classifies foods based on the rapidity of this effect on blood sugar - with fast-digesting simple carbohydrates causing a sharper increase and slower-digesting complex carbohydrates, such as whole grains, a slower one. Jenkins' research laid the scientific groundwork for subsequent low-carbohydrate diets.

In 1992, Atkins posted an update from his 1972 book, Dr. Atkins' New Diet Revolution, as well as other doctors who started to publish books based on similar principles. Through the late 1990s and early 2000s, low-carbohydrate diets became a few of the most popular diets in America. By some accounts, as much as 18% of the populace was using one kind of low-carbohydrate diet or another at the peak of their popularity. Food manufacturers and restaurant chains noted the trend since it affected their businesses. Elements of the mainstream medical community have denounced low-carbohydrate diets to be dangerous to health, like the AHA in 2001, as well as the American Kidney Fund in 2002.

Chapter 2

Popular Methods to Execute a Low Carb Diet

Low carb diets have already been popular for many years. They used to be highly controversial but have recently gained mainstream acceptance. Low carb diets tend to cause more excess weight loss than low-fat diets - at least for a while.

In addition, they improve numerous health markers, such as blood triglycerides, HDL (good) cholesterol, blood sugar levels, and blood pressure. However, various kinds of this eating pattern exist.

Listed below are 8 popular methods to execute a low carb diet.

An Average Low Carb Diet

The normal low carb diet doesn't have a set definition. It is simply known as a low carb or carb-restricted diet. This eating pattern is commonly about reduced carbs and higher in protein when compared to a typical Western diet. It usually emphasizes meats, fish, eggs, nuts, seeds, vegetables, fruits, and healthy fats.

You're designed to minimize your intake of high-carb foods like grains, potatoes, sweet drinks, and high-sugar junk food.

The recommended carb intake each day generally depends on your targets and preferences. A typical rubric may be similar to this:

100-150 grams. This stove is intended for weight maintenance or frequent high-intensity exercise. It gives room for a lot of fruit as well as some starchy foods like potatoes.

50-100 grams. This is for slow and steady weight loss or weight maintenance. There's room for a lot of fruit and veggies.

Under 50 grams. That is aimed toward quick weight loss. Eat a lot of vegetables but limit fruit intake to berries low around the glycemic index (GI).

Summary

Your typical low carb diet is a lot low in carbs and higher in protein when compared to a regular diet. The recommended carb intake depends upon specific goals and preferences.

Ketogenic Diet

The ketogenic diet is a very low-carb, high-fat diet. The purpose of a keto diet is to keep carbs so low that the body switches into a metabolic state, called *ketosis*.

In this state, your insulin levels plummet and your body releases huge amounts of essential fatty acids from its fat stores.

Many of these essential fatty acids are used in your liver, which turns them into ketones. ***Ketones*** are water-soluble substances that may cross the blood-brain barrier and offer energy to the human brain.

Then, rather than working on carbs, the human brain starts to depend on ketones. The body can produce the tiny amount of glucose still required by the human brain via a procedure called ***Gluco Neogenesis***.

Some versions of the diet even restrict protein intake because an excessive amount of protein may decrease the number of ketones you produce.

Traditionally used to take care of drug-resistant epilepsy in children, the keto diet could also have benefits for other neurological disorders and metabolic problems like type 2 diabetes.

It is also used for recognition for weight loss - even among some bodybuilders - as it's an effective way to reduce fat and will result in a major decrease in appetite.

A ketogenic diet involves high-protein, high-fat foods. Carbs are usually limited to less than 50 - and sometimes only 20-30 grams each day.

A typical keto eating pattern is known as a typical ketogenic diet (SKD).

However, you will find additional variations that involve strategically adding carbs:

Targeted ketogenic diet (TKD): In this version, you add smaller amounts of carbs around exercises.

Cyclical ketogenic diet (CKD): This kind has you take in a ketogenic diet of all days but switch to a high-carb diet for 1-2 days every week.

Summary

A ketogenic (keto) diet involves reducing carbs sufficiently to induce a metabolic state called *ketosis*. It's an extremely powerful diet to reduce fat and could protect against many diseases.

Low-Carb, High-Fat (LCHF)

LCHF means *"low-carb, high-fat."* It's a reasonably standard very-low carb diet but with a much greater emphasis on whole, unprocessed foods.

It focuses mostly on meats, seafood, eggs, healthy fats, vegetables, milk products, nut products, and berries.

The recommended carb intake on this diet can range between 20-100 grams each day.

Summary

The **LCHF diet** is a very low carb eating pattern that focuses mostly on whole, unprocessed foods.

Low Carb Paleo Diet

The *paleo diet* happens to be among the world's most popular means of eating. It encourages eating food that originates from the ***Paleolithic era*** - before the agricultural and industrial revolutions.

According to paleo proponents, time for the diet of the prehistoric ancestors should improve health because humans allegedly evolved and adapted to eating such foods. Several small studies also show a paleo diet could cause fat loss, reduce blood sugars, and improve risk factors for cardiovascular disease.

A paleo diet isn't low carb by definition but is commonly so used. It emphasizes meats, fish, seafood, eggs, vegetables, fruits, tubers, nuts, and seeds. A strict paleo diet eliminates processed food items, added sugar, grains, legumes, and milk products. There are many other popular versions, like the primal blueprint and perfect health diets. Most of them tend to be lower in carbs when compared to a typical Western diet.

Summary

The paleo diet involves eating unprocessed foods which were likely common and peculiar to your Paleolithic ancestors. Without strictly low-carb, it could be modified to match such a lifestyle.

The Atkins Diet

The Atkins diet is the best-known low carb diet program. It involves reducing all high-carb foods while eating just as much protein and fat as desired.

<u>The dietary plan is divided into four phases:</u>

Phase 1: *Induction-* Eat below 20 grams of carbs each day for 14 days.

Phase 2: *Balancing-* Slowly add more nuts, low carb vegetables, and fruit.

Phase 3: *Fine-tuning-* Whenever you get near your body weight goal, add more carbs until your body weight loss becomes slower.

Phase 4: *Maintenance-* Eat as many healthy carbs as the body tolerates without gaining back the weight you lost.

The Atkins diet was originally demonized, but current research indicates it's both effective and safe so long as fiber intake is adequate. The dietary plan continues to be popular today.

Summary

The Atkins diet continues to be popular for over 40 years. It is a 4-phase, low carb eating pattern which allows you to take a lot of fat and protein.

Eco-Atkins

A diet plan termed Eco-Atkins is a vegan version of the Atkins diet. It offers plant foods and things that are saturated in protein and/or fat, such as gluten, soy, nuts, and plant oils. About 25% of its calories result from carbs, 30% from protein, and 45% from fat.

Therefore, it's higher in carbs when compared to a typical Atkins diet - but much lower when compared to a typical vegan diet. One six-month report showed an Eco-Atkins diet caused more excess weight loss and greater improvement in cardiovascular disease risk factors when compared to a high-carb vegetarian diet plan.

Summary

The Eco-Atkins diet can be a vegan version of the Atkins diet. While higher in carbs when compared to a typical Atkins diet, it's still very low carb in comparison to most vegetarian and vegan diets.

Zero-Carb

Some people prefer to remove all carbs using their diet. That is called a zero-carb diet and has only animal foods. People who follow a zero-carb diet eat meat, fish, eggs, and animal fats like butter and lard. A few of them also add salt and spices.

You will find no recent studies that show a zero-carb diet to be safe. Only 1 research study - from 1930 - exists, where two men ate only meat and organs for a year but seemed to maintain a healthy body.

A zero-carb diet is without some important nutrients, such as vitamin C and fiber. Because of this, it is generally not recommended.

Summary

Some people follow a zero-carb diet, which excludes all plant foods. No quality studies have already been done on this eating pattern, which is usually discouraged.

Low carb Mediterranean Diet

The Mediterranean diet is quite popular, especially among medical researchers. It is based on the original foods of Mediterranean countries earlier in the 20th century. Studies show that diet can help prevent cardiovascular disease, breast cancer, and type 2 diabetes.

A low carb Mediterranean eating pattern is modeled following its similar diet but limits higher-carb foods like whole grains.

Unlike a normal low carb diet, it emphasizes more fatty fish rather than red meat and much more extra virgin olive oil rather than fats like butter. A low carb Mediterranean diet could be better for cardiovascular disease prevention than other low carb diets, although this must be confirmed in studies.

Summary

A low carb Mediterranean diet is compared to a normal low carb diet. However, it has more fish and further virgin olive oil. If you're likely to get one of these low carb diets, choose a plan that suits your way of life, food preferences, and personal health goals. What works for one person might not work for another, therefore the best diet for you personally may be the one you can stick to.

Does it Aid Weight Loss?

A low carb diet limits carbohydrates - such as those in grains, starchy fruit, and veggies - and emphasizes foods saturated in protein and fat. Various kinds of low carb diets exist. Each diet has varying restrictions on the types and levels of carbohydrates you can eat.

Purpose

A low carb diet is normally used for slimming down. Some low carb diets may have health advantages beyond weight loss, such as reducing risk factors connected with type 2 diabetes and metabolic syndrome.

Why choose a low carb diet?

You may choose a low carb diet because you:

- Need a diet that restricts certain carbs to help you lose weight.
- Want to improve your overall feeding habits.
- Benefit from the types and levels of foods featured in low carb diets.
- Consult with your doctor before starting any weight-loss diet, particularly if you might have any health issues, such as diabetes or cardiovascular disease.

Diet Details

As the name says, a low carb diet restricts the sort and amount of carbohydrates you take in. Carbohydrates are a kind of calorie-providing macronutrient in many foods and beverages. Carbohydrates could be simple or complex. They can be further classified as easy processed (table sugar), simple natural (lactose in milk and fructose in fruit), complex refined (bleached flour), and complex natural (whole grains or beans).

Common resources of naturally occurring carbohydrates have:

- Grains.
- Fruits.
- Vegetables.
- Milk.
- Nuts.
- Seeds.
- Legumes (beans, lentils, peas).

Food manufacturers also add refined carbohydrates to processed food items using sugar or bleached flour. Types of foods that contain complex carbohydrates are white bread and pasta, cookies, cake, candy, and sugar-sweetened sodas and drinks.

The body uses carbohydrates as its main fuel source. Complex carbohydrates (starches) are broken into simple sugars during digestion. They're then absorbed into the bloodstream, where they're referred to as blood sugar levels (glucose). Generally, natural complex carbohydrates are digested more slowly plus they have less influence on blood glucose. Natural complex carbohydrates provide bulk and serve other body functions beyond fuel. Rising degrees of glucose levels trigger your body and release insulin. Insulin helps glucose enter your cells. Some glucose can be used by the body for energy, fueling all your activities, be it taking a jog or just breathing. Extra glucose is normally kept in your liver, and muscles along with other cells for later use or is changed into fat.

The theory behind the low carb diet is the fact that decreasing carbs lowers insulin amounts, which causes your body to burn stored fat for energy and ultimately results in weight loss.

Chapter 3

Typical Foods for a Low Carb Diet

Generally, a low carb diet targets proteins, including meat, chicken, fish, and eggs, plus some non-starchy vegetables. A low carb diet generally excludes or limits most grains, legumes, fruits, bread, sweets, pasta and starchy vegetables, and sometimes nuts and seeds. Some low carb weight loss programs allow smaller amounts of fruits, vegetables, and whole grains.

A regular limit of 0.7 to 2 ounces (20 to 60 grams) of carbohydrates is typical having a low carb diet. These levels of carbohydrates provide 80 to 240 calories. Some low carb diets greatly restrict carbs through the initial phase of the dietary plan and gradually increase the number of allowed carbs.

On the other hand, the Dietary Guidelines for Americans recommends that carbohydrates constitute 45 to 65 percent of the total day-by-day calorie intake. If you eat 2,000 calories each day, you would have to eat between 900 and 1,300 calories per day from carbohydrates.

Results

Weight Loss

A lot of people can slim down if they restrict the number of calories consumed and increase exercise levels. To reduce 1 to at least one 1.5 pounds (0.5 to 0.7 kilogram) weekly, you require to lessen your day-by-day calories by 500 to 750 calories.

Low carb diets can lead to greater short-term fat loss than do low-fat diets. But most studies have discovered that at one or two years, the advantages of a low carb diet aren't obvious. A 2015 review discovered that higher protein, low-carbohydrate diets may provide a slight advantage with regards to weight loss and lack of fat mass weighed against a standard protein diet.

Cutting calories and carbs may not be the only reason behind the weight loss. Some studies also show that you might shed a few pounds because the spare protein and fat keep you feeling full longer, which can help you eat less.

Other Health Advantages

Low carb diets can help prevent or improve serious health issues, such as metabolic syndrome, diabetes, high blood pressure, and coronary disease. Nearly every diet that can help you lose weight can reduce and reverse risk factors for coronary disease and diabetes. Most weight-loss diets - not only low carb diets - may improve blood cholesterol or blood sugar, at least temporarily.

Low carb diets may improve high-density lipoprotein (HDL) cholesterol and triglyceride values slightly a lot more than moderate-carb diets. This may be due not only to how many carbs you take but also to the grade of your additional food choices. Lean protein (fish, chicken, legumes), healthy fats (monounsaturated and polyunsaturated), and unprocessed carbs - such as whole grains, legumes, vegetables, fruits, and low-fat milk products - are usually healthier choices.

A report from the American Heart Association, the American College of Cardiology as well as the Obesity Society figured there is not enough evidence to state whether most low-carbohydrate diets provide heart-healthy benefits.

Risks

In case you suddenly and drastically cut carbs, you might experience some temporary health effects, including:

- Headache.
- Bad breath.
- Weakness.
- Muscle cramps.
- Fatigue.
- Skin rash.
- Constipation or diarrhea.

Furthermore, some diets restrict carbohydrate intake a lot, in the long run, they can cause vitamin or mineral deficiencies, bone loss, and gastrointestinal disturbances and could increase the risks of varied chronic diseases.

Because low carb diets might not provide necessary nutrients, these diets aren't recommended as a way of fat loss for pre-teens and high schoolers. Their growing bodies need the nutrients in whole grains, fruits & vegetables.

Severely restricting carbohydrates to significantly less than 0.7 ounces (20 grams) every day can lead to an activity called **ketosis**. *Ketosis* occurs when you do not have enough sugar (glucose) for energy, which means that your body reduces placed fat, causing ketones to develop in you. Side effects from ketosis range from nausea, headache, mental and physical fatigue, and bad breath.

It's not clear the type of possible long-term health threats a low carb diet may pose because most clinical tests have lasted significantly less than a year. Some health experts think that if you take in huge amounts of fat and protein from animal sources, your threat of cardiovascular disease or particular cancers could increase.

In case you follow a low-carbohydrate diet that's higher in fat and perhaps higher in protein, it is critical to choose foods with healthy unsaturated fats and healthy proteins. Limit foods containing saturated and trans fats, such as meat, high-fat milk products, and prepared crackers and pastries.

A Low carb Meal Plan and Menu to boost Your Health

A low carb diet is a diet that restricts carbohydrates, such as those in sugary foods, pasta, and bread. It is saturated in protein, fat and healthy vegetables.

There are various types of low carb diets, and studies also show they can cause weight loss and improve health.

This is an in-depth meal arranged for a low carb diet. It explains what things to eat, and what things to avoid and has a sample low carb menu for one week.

Low carb Feeding - The Fundamentals

Your meal choices rely on a couple of things, including how healthy you are, how much you exercise, and how much weight you must lose.

Think about this meal plan as an overall guideline, not at all something written in stone.

Eat: Meat, fish, eggs, vegetables, fruit, nuts, seeds, high-fat dairy, fats, healthy oils, and perhaps even some tubers and non-gluten grains.

Don't eat: Sugar, HFCS, wheat, seed oils, trans fats, "diet" and low-fat products, and ready-made foods.

Foods to avoid

You need to avoid these six food groups and nutrients:

Sugar: Carbonated drinks, fruit drinks, agave, chocolate, ice cream, and several other products which contain added sugar.

Processed grains: Wheat, rice, barley, rye, bread, cereal, and pasta.

Trans fats: Hydrogenated or partially hydrogenated oils.

Diet and low-fat products: Many milk products, cereals or crackers are fat-reduced but contain added sugar.

Ready-made foods: If it seems to be produced in a factory, don't eat them.

Starchy vegetables: It's better to limit starchy vegetables in what you eat if you're carrying out a very low carb diet.

You need to read ingredient lists on foods labeled as health foods.

Foods to Eat

You must base your daily diet on these real, unprocessed, low carb foods.

Meat: Beef, lamb, pork, chicken as well as others; grass-fed is most beneficial.

Fish: Salmon, trout, haddock, and many more; wild-caught fish is most beneficial.

Eggs: Omega-3-enriched or pastured eggs are best.

Vegetables: Spinach, broccoli, cauliflower, carrots, and many more.

Fruits: Apples, oranges, pears, blueberries, strawberries.

Nut products and seeds: Almonds, walnuts, sunflower seeds, etc.

High-fat dairy: Cheese, butter, heavy cream, yogurt.

Fats and oils: Coconut oil, butter, lard, olive oil, and fish oil.

If you want to shed weight, be cautious with cheese and nut products, as it's simple to overeat them. Don't eat even more than one little bit of fruit each day.

Foods You Can Eat

If you're healthy, active, and don't have to slim down, you can eat some more carbs.

Tubers: Potatoes, sweet potatoes, plus some others.

Unrefined grains: Brown rice, oats, quinoa, and many more.

Legumes: Lentils, black beans, pinto beans, etc. (when you can tolerate them).

<u>What's more, you could take the following in moderation, if you'd like:</u>

Chocolates: Choose organic brands with at least 70% of cocoa.

Wine: Choose dry wines without added sugar or carbs.

Dark chocolate is usually saturated in antioxidants and could provide health advantages if you must eat them, eat moderately. However, remember that both chocolates and alcohol will hinder your progress if you eat/drink them excessively.

- Beverages
- Coffee
- Tea
- Water
- Sugar-free carbonated beverages, like water.

Low carb Menu for a Week

This is an example menu for one week on a low carb diet program.

It provides significantly less than 50 grams of total carbs each day. However, if you're healthy and active you can eat slightly more carbs.

Monday

Breakfast: Omelet with various vegetables, fried in butter or coconut oil.

Lunch: Grass-fed yogurt with blueberries and a small number of almonds.

Supper: Bunless cheeseburger, served with vegetables and salsa sauce.

Tuesday

Breakfast: Bacon and eggs.

Lunch: Leftover burgers and veggies from the previous night.

Supper: Salmon with butter and vegetables.

Wednesday

Breakfast: Eggs and vegetables, fried in butter or coconut oil.

Lunch: Shrimp salad with some olive oil.

Supper: Grilled chicken with vegetables.

Thursday

Breakfast: Omelet with various vegetables, fried in butter or coconut oil.

Lunch: Smoothie with coconut milk, berries, almonds, and protein powder.

Supper: Steak and veggies.

Friday

Breakfast: Bacon and eggs.

Lunch: Chicken salad with some olive oil.

Supper: Pork chops with vegetables.

Saturday

Breakfast: Omelet with various veggies.

Lunch: Grass-fed yogurt with berries, coconut flakes, and a small number of walnuts.

Supper: Meatballs with vegetables.

Sunday

Breakfast: Bacon and eggs.

Lunch: Smoothie with coconut milk, a dash of heavy cream, chocolate-flavored protein powder, and berries.

Supper: Grilled chicken wings with some raw spinach privately.

Have a lot of low carb vegetables in what you eat. If your goal is to stay under 50 grams of carbs each day, there is room for a lot of veggies and one fruit each day.

Again, if you're healthy, lean, and active, you can have some tubers like potatoes and sweet potatoes, as well as some healthy grains like oats.

Healthy, Low carb Snacks

There is no health reason to eat more than three meals each day, but if you get hungry between meals, below are a few healthy, easy-to-prepare, low carb snacks that may fill you up:

- A bit of fruit.
- Full-fat yogurt.
- A couple of hard-boiled eggs.
- Baby carrots.
- Leftovers from the prior night.
- A small number of nuts.
- Some cheese and meat.
- Going out to restaurants.

For the most part restaurants, it's simple enough to make meals low carb friendly.

- Order meat- or fish-based main dish.
- Drink only water rather than sugary soda or juice.
- Get surplus vegetables rather than a loaf of bread, potatoes, or rice.

A simple Low carb grocery list

An excellent rule is to look in the aisle of the store, where the whole foods can be found.

Focusing on entire foods can make your diet plan a thousand times better than the typical Western diet.

Organic and grass-fed foods are also popular choices and frequently considered healthier, but they're typically more costly.

Try to pick the least processed option that still fits into your budget.

- Meat (beef, lamb, pork, chicken, bacon)
- Fish (fatty fish like salmon is most beneficial)
- Eggs (choose omega-3 enriched or pastured eggs when you can)

- Butter
- Coconut oil
- Lard
- Olive oil
- Cheese
- Heavy cream
- Sour cream
- Yogurt (full-fat, unsweetened)
- Blueberries (fresh or frozen)
- Nuts
- Olives
- More fresh vegetables (greens, peppers, onions, etc.)
- Frozen vegetables (broccoli, carrots, various mixes)
- Condiments (sea salt, pepper, garlic, mustard, etc.)

Clear your pantry of most unhealthy temptations when you can, such as chips, candy, ice cream, sodas, juices, bread, cereals, and baking ingredients like refined flour and sugar.

Bottom Line

Low carb diets restrict carbs, such as those in sugary and processed food items, pasta, and bakery. They're saturated in protein, fat and healthy vegetables.

Studies show they can cause weight loss and improve health.

The aforementioned meal plan offers you the fundamentals of healthy, low carb eating.

Chapter 4

Best Low carb Vegetables

Vegetables are low in calories but abundant with vitamins, minerals along with other important nutrients. In addition, most are low in carbs and saturated in fiber, making them perfect for low carb diets.

The definition of the low carb diet varies widely. The majority are under 150 grams of carbs each day, and some exceed only 20 grams each day. Whether you're on a low carb diet or not, eating more vegetables is a good idea.

This is a set of the 21 best low carb vegetables relating to your diet.

Bell Peppers

Bell peppers, also called *sweet peppers or capsicums*, are incredibly nutritious. They contain antioxidants called carotenoids that could reduce inflammation, decrease cancer risk, and protect cholesterol and fats from oxidative damage.

One cup (149 grams) of chopped red pepper contains 9 grams of carbs, 3 of which are fiber. It offers 93% of the

Reference Daily Intake (RDI) for vitamin A and an impressive 317% in the **RDI** for vitamin C, which is often lacking on very low carb diets.

Green, orange, and yellow bell peppers have similar nutrient profiles, although their antioxidant contents can vary greatly.

Summary

Bell peppers are anti-inflammatory and saturated in vitamins A and C. They contain 6 grams of digestible (net) carbs per portion.

Broccoli

Broccoli is a genuine superfood. It's a family of the cruciferous vegetable family, which has kale, Brussels sprouts, radishes, and cabbage.

Studies also show that broccoli may decrease insulin resistance in type 2 diabetics. It is also considered to protect against various kinds of cancer, including prostate cancer. One cup (91 grams) of raw broccoli contains 6 grams of carbs, 2 of which are fiber.

In addition, it provides more than 100% of the RDI for vitamins C and K.

Summary

Broccoli contains 4 grams of digestible carbs per portion. It's saturated in vitamins C and K and could reduce insulin resistance and help to prevent cancer.

Asparagus

Asparagus is a delicious spring vegetable. One cup (180 grams) of cooked asparagus contains 8 grams of carbs, 4 of which are fiber. It is also a good way to obtain vitamins A, C, and K (9). Test-tube studies have discovered that asparagus can prevent the growth of various kinds of cancer, and studies in mice suggest it could support protect brain health.

Summary

Asparagus contains 4 grams of digestible carbs per portion. It's an excellent source of many vitamins and could prevent some types of cancer.

Mushrooms

Mushrooms are really low in carbs. A one-cup (70-gram) serving of raw, white mushrooms contains just 2 grams of carbs, 1 of which is dietary fiber (15). What's more, they are shown to possess strong anti-inflammatory properties.

In a report on men with metabolic syndrome, eating 3.5 ounces (100 grams) of white mushrooms for 16 weeks resulted in significant improvements in antioxidant and anti-inflammatory markers.

Summary

Mushrooms contain 1 gram of digestible carbs per portion. They can reduce inflammation in people who have metabolic syndrome.

Zucchini

Zucchini is a favorite vegetable and the most frequent kind of summer squash. Summer squash is long with soft skin that may be eaten. On the other hand, winter squash will come in several shapes, comes with an inedible rind, and is higher in carbs than summer varieties.

One cup (124 grams) of raw zucchini contains 4 grams of carbs, 1 of which is usually fiber. It's an excellent way to obtain vitamin C, providing 35% of the RDI per portion. Yellow Italian squash and other styles of summer squash have carb counts and nutrient profiles much like zucchini.

Summary

Zucchini and other styles of summer squash contain 3 grams of digestible carbs per portion and are saturated in vitamin C.

Spinach

Spinach is a leafy green vegetable that delivers major health advantages. Researchers report that it can reduce harm to DNA. In addition, it protects heart health and may reduce the threat of common eye diseases like cataracts and macular degeneration.

Also, it's loaded with several minerals and vitamins. One cup (180 grams) of cooked spinach provides a lot more than 10 occasions the RDI for vitamin K (22).

Spinach can be low in carbs; however, the carbs are more concentrated as the leaves are cooked down and lose their nutrients.

For example, one glass of cooked spinach contains 7 grams of carbs with 4 grams of fiber, whereas one glass of raw spinach contains 1 gram of carbs with almost 1 gram of fiber (22, 23).

Summary

Cooked spinach contains 3 grams of digestible carbs per portion, is very saturated in vitamin K and helps protect the heart and eye health.

Avocados

Avocados certainly are a unique and delicious food. Although technically a fruit, avocados are usually eaten as vegetables. They're also saturated in fat and contain hardly any digestible carbs.

A one-cup (150-gram) serving of chopped avocados has 13 grams of carbs, 10 of which are fiber (24). Avocados are also rich in oleic acid, a kind of monounsaturated fat that has beneficial effects on health. Small studies have discovered that avocados might help lower LDL cholesterol and triglyceride levels.

They're also an excellent way to obtain vitamin C, folate, and potassium. Although avocados are a fairly high-calorie food, they might be beneficial for weight loss. In one report, overweight people who had half an avocado in their lunch reported feeling fuller and had less desire to eat over another five hours.

Summary

Avocados provide 3 grams of net carbs per portion. They enhance feelings of fullness and so are saturated in heart-healthy fat and fiber.

Cauliflower

Cauliflower is among the most versatile and popular low carb vegetables. It has a very mild taste and may be used as an alternative for potatoes, grain as well as other higher-carb foods. One cup (100 grams) of raw cauliflower contains 5 grams of carbs, 3 of which are fiber. It is also saturated in vitamin K and 77% in the RDI for vitamin C (28).

Like other cruciferous vegetables, it's connected with a reduced threat of cardiovascular disease and cancer.

Summary

Cauliflower contains 2 grams of digestible carbs per portion. Also, it is saturated in vitamins K and C and could help prevent cardiovascular disease and cancer.

Green Beans

Green beans are occasionally known as snap beans or string beans. They are a part of the legume family, along with beans and lentils. However, they have got considerably fewer carbs than most legumes.

A one-cup (125-gram) serving of cooked green beans contains 10 grams of carbs, 4 of which are fibers. They're saturated in chlorophyll, which studies suggest can prevent cancer.

Furthermore, they contain *carotenoids*, that are connected with improved brain function during aging.

Summary

Green beans contain 6 grams of digestible carbs per portion, as well as antioxidants that might help prevent cancer and protect the mind.

Lettuce

Lettuce is one of the lowest-carb vegetables around. One cup (47 grams) of lettuce contains 2 grams of carbs, 1 of which is fiber (34).

With regards to the type, it could also be considered a good way to obtain certain vitamins. For example, romaine along with other dark-green varieties is abundant with vitamins A, C, and K.

They're also saturated in *folate*. **Folate** helps decrease degrees of *homocysteine*; a compound associated with an increased threat of heart disease.

One research in 37 women showed that eating foods saturated in folate for five weeks reduced homocysteine levels by 13%, in comparison to a low-folate diet.

Summary

Lettuce contains 1 gram of digestible carbs per portion. It's saturated in some vitamins, including folate, which might reduce cardiovascular disease risk.

Garlic

Garlic is well known because of its beneficial effects on immune function. Studies have discovered that it could boost resistance to the normal cold and decrease blood pressure. Although the high-carb vegetable by weight, the total amount typically consumed in a single sitting is quite low because of its strong taste and aroma. One clove (3 grams) of garlic contains 1 gram of carbs, a part which is fiber.

Summary

Garlic contains 1 gram of digestible carbs per clove. It could reduce blood pressure and improve immune function.

Kale

Kale is a trendy vegetable that's also extremely nutrient-dense. It's packed with antioxidants, including *quercetin* and *kaempferol.*

These have been proven to reduce blood pressure and could also prevent cardiovascular disease, type 2 diabetes as well as other diseases.

One cup (67 grams) of raw kale contains 7 grams of carbs, one of which is certainly fiber. In addition, it has an impressive 206% **RDI** for vitamin A and 134% the **RDI** for vitamin C. A higher intake of vitamin C has been proven to boost immune function and raise the skin's ability to fight damaging free radicals, which may speed up aging.

Summary

Kale contains 6 grams of digestible carbs per portion. It's saturated in antioxidants and has a lot more than 100% of the RDI for vitamins A and C.

Cucumbers

Cucumbers are lower in carbs and incredibly refreshing. One cup (104 grams) of chopped cucumber contains 4 grams of carbs, significantly less than 1 gram which is normally fiber. Although cucumbers aren't high in vitamins or nutrients, they have a compound called *cucurbitacin E*, which might have beneficial effects on health.

Results from test-tube and animal studies suggest they have anti-cancer and anti-inflammatory houses and could protect brain health.

Summary

Cucumbers contain slightly below 4 grams of digestible carbs per portion. They aid the prevention of cancer and support brain health.

Brussels Sprouts

Brussels sprouts are another tasty cruciferous vegetable. A half-cup (78-gram) serving of cooked Brussels sprouts contains 6 grams of carbs, 2 of which are fiber (50).

In addition, it provides 80% of the *RDI* for vitamin C and 137% of the *RDI* for vitamin K. Also, controlled human studies claim that eating Brussels sprouts may reduce risk factors for cancer, including cancer of the colon.

Summary

Brussels sprouts contain 4 grams of digestible carbs per portion. They're saturated in vitamins C and K and could reduce cancer risk.

Celery

Celery is low in digestible carbs. A one-cup (101-gram) serving of chopped celery contains 3 grams of carbs, 2 of which are dietary fiber. It's an excellent way to obtain vitamin K, providing 37% of the **RDI**.

In addition, it has *luteolin*, an antioxidant that can prevent and help treat cancer.

Summary

Celery provides 1 gram of digestible carbs per portion. Also, it contains luteolin, which might have anti-cancer properties.

Tomatoes

Tomatoes have several impressive health advantages. Like avocados, they may be technically fruits but are usually consumed as vegetables. They're also low in digestible carbs. One cup (149 grams) of cherry tomatoes contains 6 grams of carbs, 2 of which are fiber. Tomatoes are a great way to obtain vitamins A, C, and K.

Furthermore, they're saturated in potassium, which may help reduce blood pressure and decrease stroke risk. They've been proven to fortify the endothelial cells that line your arteries, and their high lycopene content can help prevent prostate cancer.

Cooking tomatoes increases lycopene content, and adding fats such as olive oil during cooking has been shown to improve its absorption.

Summary

Tomatoes contain 4 grams of digestible carbs per portion and are saturated in vitamins and potassium. They might support protecting heart health and reducing cancer risk.

Radishes

Radishes are Brassica vegetables having a sharp, peppery taste. One cup (116 grams) of raw sliced radishes contains 4 grams of carbs, 2 of which are fiber. They're fairly saturated in vitamin C, providing 29% of the RDI per portion.

Also, radishes may decrease the threat of breast cancer in postmenopausal women by modifying the kind of body that metabolizes estrogen.

Summary

Radishes contain 2 grams of digestible carbs per portion and may lessen the chance of breast cancer in older women.

Onions

Onions are a pungent, nutritious vegetable. Although they are fairly saturated in carbs by weight, they may be consumed in smaller amounts for their robust flavor.

A half-cup (58 grams) of sliced raw onions contains 6 grams of carbs, 1 of which is fibers. Onions are saturated in the antioxidant quercetin, which might lower blood pressure.

One review in overweight and obese women with **polycystic ovary syndrome (PCOS)** discovered that eating red onions reduced *LDL cholesterol levels.*

Summary Onions contain 5 grams of digestible carbs per portion and may support lower blood pressure and LDL cholesterol levels.

Eggplant

Eggplant is a common vegetable in lots of Italian and Asian dishes. A one-cup (99-gram) serving of chopped, cooked eggplant contains 8 grams of carbs, 2 of which are fiber. It's not abundant in most vitamins or minerals, but animal research suggests eggplant can help lower cholesterol and improve other markers of heart health.

In addition, it contains an antioxidant referred to as *nasunin* in the purple pigment of its skin. Researchers have reported that *nasunin* helps reduce free radicals and could protect brain health.

Summary

Eggplant contains 6 grams of digestible carbs per portion and may support protect heart and brain health.

Cabbage

Cabbage has some impressive health advantages. Like a cruciferous vegetable, it could help reduce the chance of certain cancers, including esophageal and stomach cancer. One cup (89 grams) of chopped raw cabbage contains 5 grams of carbs, 3 of which are fiber.

In addition, it provides 54% of the RDI for vitamin C and 85% of the RDI for vitamin K.

Summary

Cabbage contains 2 grams of digestible carbs per portion. It's saturated in vitamins C and K and could reduce the threat of certain cancers.

Artichokes

Artichokes are delicious and nutritious. One medium-sized globe artichoke (120 grams) contains 14 grams of carbs.

However, 10 grams result from fiber, rendering it surprisingly low in digestible (net) carbs. A portion of the fiber is *inulin*, which acts as a prebiotic that feeds healthy gut bacteria.

Also, artichokes may protect heart health. In a single study, when people who have high cholesterol drank artichoke juice, they experienced a decrease in inflammatory markers and improvement in blood vessel function.

Summary

Artichokes contain 4 grams of digestible carbs per portion and could improve gut and heart health. Numerous tasty vegetables may be had on a low carb diet.

Not only is it low in carbs and calories, they could lower your risk of diseases and improve your current health and well-being.

Chapter 5

Myths About Low Carb Diets

There's a large amount of misinformation about low carb diets. Some say that it's the perfect human diet, while some contemplate it as an unsustainable and potentially harmful fad.

Listed below are common myths about low carb diets.

They're just a fad

The word *"crash diet"* was used for crash weight loss diets that enjoyed short-term popularity. Today, it's often misused for diets that don't have common cultural acceptance, including low carb diets.

However, a low carb method of eating has been shown to work in over 20 scientific tests. Plus, it's been popular for many years. The first Atkins' book was published in 1972, five years before the first group of low-fat dietary guidelines in the U/S.

Looking back, the first low carb book was published by William Banting in 1863 and was wildly popular at that time. Taking into consideration the long-term and scientifically proven success of low carb diets, dismissing this manner of eating like a fad seems far-fetched.

Summary

Crash diets enjoy short-term popularity and success. On the other hand, the low carb diet's been around for decades and it is supported by over 20 high-quality human studies.

Hard to stick with

Opponents often declare that low carb diets are unsustainable because they restrict common food groups. This is thought to result in feelings of deprivation, causing newbies to abandon the dietary plan and regain weight.

Still, consider that all diets restrict something - some certain food groups or macronutrients, others calories. Carrying out a low carb diet has been shown to lessen appetite to enable you to eat until satisfied but still slim down.

In contrast, on the calorie-restricted diet, you're less inclined to eat until you're fully satisfied and could be hungry regularly - that is unsustainable for many people.

Scientific evidence does not support that low carb diets are harder to adhere to than additional diets.

Summary

Science does not support the theory that low carb diets are hard to adhere to. They enable you to eat until you're satisfied while still slimming down, which is even more sustainable than calorie-restricted diets.

A lot of the weight loss comes from water

The body stores a lot of carbs in your muscles and liver. It runs on the storage type of glucose referred to as glycogen, which supplies the body with glucose between meals. Stored glycogen in your liver and muscles will bind some water. Whenever you cut carbs, your glycogen stores decrease, and also you lose a lot of water weight.

Also, low carb diets result in drastically reduced insulin levels, causing your kidneys to shed excess sodium and water. Therefore, low carb diets result in a considerable and almost immediate decrease in water weight.

This is used as a disagreement against this method of eating, and it's claimed that the only reason behind its weight loss advantage may be the decrease in water weight.

However, studies also show that low carb diets also reduce surplus fat - especially from the liver and abdominal region where harmful stomach fat is situated. For instance, one 6-week study on low carb diets showed that participants lost 7.5 pounds (3.4 kg) of fat but gained 2.4 pounds (1.1 kg) of muscles.

Summary

People who eat a low carb diet shed excess water but also surplus fat, especially from the liver and abdominal region.

Harmful to the heart

Low carb diets tend to be saturated in cholesterol and fat, including saturated fat. Because of this, many people say that their blood cholesterol increases and also increases the risk of heart disease. However, some studies claim that neither dietary cholesterol nor saturated fat has any significant influence on your threat of cardiovascular disease.

Most of all, low carb diets may improve many important cardiovascular disease risk factors by:

- considerably decreasing blood triglycerides,
- increasing HDL (good) cholesterol,
- lowering blood pressure,
- decreasing insulin resistance, which reduces blood sugar levels and insulin amounts,
- reducing inflammation.

What's more, levels of LDL (bad) cholesterol generally don't increase. Plus, these particles tend to differ from harmful, small, dense shapes to larger ones - an activity associated with a lower life expectancy risk of cardiovascular disease.

Still, consider that these studies mostly take a look at averages. A lot of people may experience major increases in LDL (bad) cholesterol over a low carb diet. If this is your case, you can adjust your low carb diet to get your levels down.

Summary

There is no evidence that dietary cholesterol and saturated fat cause harm, and studies on low carb diets show they improve several key risk factors for cardiovascular disease.

They work because people eat fewer calories

Many people say that the real reason people shed weight on low carb diets is because of reduced calorie consumption. That is true but doesn't tell the complete story.

The main fat loss benefit of low carb diets is the fact that weight loss occurs automatically. People feel so full they end up eating less food without counting calories or controlling portions.

Low carb diets also tend to be saturated in protein, which boosts metabolism, causing a huge increase in the number of calories you burn. Plus, low carb diets aren't always about slimming down. They're also effective against certain health conditions, such as metabolic syndrome, type 2 diabetes, and epilepsy. In such cases, medical benefits exceed reduced calorie consumption.

Summary

Though low carb diets cause reduced calorie consumption, the fact that happens subconsciously is a big benefit. Low carb diets also aid metabolic health.

They lessen your consumption of healthy plant foods

A low carb diet is not a no-carb. It's a myth that cutting carbs implies that you need to eat fewer plant foods.

You can eat huge amounts of vegetables, berries, nuts, and seeds without exceeding 50 grams of carbs each day. What's more, eating 100-150 grams of carbs each day continues to be considered low-carb. This gives room for some bits of fruit each day and even smaller amounts of healthy starches like potatoes and oats. It's possible and sustainable to eat low carb on a vegetarian or vegan diet.

Summary

You can eat a lot of plant foods despite having an extremely low carbohydrate intake. Vegetables, berries, nuts, and seeds are types of healthy plant foods which are low in carbs.

Ketosis is a dangerous metabolic state

There's a lot of confusion surrounding ketosis. When you eat fewer carbs - such as less than 50 grams each day - your insulin amounts go down and lots of fat is released from your fat cells. When your liver gets flooded with essential fatty acids, it starts to convert them into ketone bodies, or ketones.

These are substances that cross the blood-brain barrier, supplying energy to the human brain during starvation or when you don't eat carbs. Many people confuse *"ketosis"* with *"ketoacidosis."* The latter can be a dangerous metabolic state that mainly happens in unmanaged type 1 diabetes. It involves your blood getting flooded with massive levels of ketones, enough to carefully turn your blood acidic.

Ketoacidosis is an extremely serious condition and may be fatal. However, that is completely unrelated to the ketosis effect of a low carb diet, which is a healthy metabolic state.

For instance, ketosis has been proven to have therapeutic effects in epilepsy and has been studied for treating cancer and brain diseases like Alzheimer's.

Summary

A very low carb diet results in the beneficial metabolic state of ketosis. This is not like *ketoacidosis*, which is dangerous but merely happens in unmanaged type 1 diabetes.

The human brain needs carbs to operate

Many people think that the human brain cannot function without dietary carbs.

It's claimed that carbs are the required fuel for the human brain and that it requires about 130 grams of carbs each day. That is partly true. Some cells in the human brain cannot use any fuel besides carbs through glucose. Yet, other areas of the human brain work well with using ketones.

If carbs are reduced sufficiently to induce ketosis, a large part of the human brain stops using glucose and starts using ketones instead. That said, despite having high blood ketone levels, some elements of your brain however need glucose. That's where a metabolic pathway called *gluconeogenesis* comes in. Once you don't eat carbs, the body - mostly your liver - can make glucose out of protein and byproducts of fat metabolism.

Therefore, due to ketosis and gluconeogenesis, you don't need dietary carbs - at least not for fueling the human brain. Following the initial adaptation phase, many people report feeling with brain function over a low carb diet.

Summary
On the low carb diet, an integral part of your brain may use ketones for fuel. The body then produces the tiny glucose that other areas of the human brain need.

They destroy physical performance

Most athletes eat a high-carb diet, and several people think that carbs are crucial for physical performance. Reducing carbs Adds to reduced performance initially.

However, normally, this is only temporary. Normally it takes your body some time to adjust to losing fat rather than carbs. Many studies display that low carb diets are best for physical performance, especially endurance exercise, as long you give yourself a couple weeks to adjust to the dietary plan.

More studies indicate that low carb diets benefit muscle tissue and strength.

Summary

Low carb diets aren't detrimental to physical performance for many people. However, normally it takes a couple weeks for the body to adapt. Low carb diets can have powerful health advantages. They're quite effective for those who have obesity, metabolic syndrome, and type 2 diabetes, however, they're not for everybody. Nonetheless, many common notions about low carb eating are untrue.

Common Low carb Mistakes (and how to avoid them)

While low carb diets have become popular, it's also easy to make mistakes with them. Numerous stumbling blocks may lead to undesirable effects and sub-optimal results. To enjoy all the metabolic great things about low carb diets, merely reducing the carbs is not enough.

Listed below are the most typical low carb mistakes - and how to prevent them.

Eating Too Many Carbs

Since there is no strict definition of a low carb diet, anything under 100-150 grams each day is normally considered low-carb. This amount happens to be more than the typical Western diet. You might achieve great results in this carb range, as long you eat unprocessed, real foods. But if you wish to enter ketosis - which is vital for any ketogenic diet - then this level of intake could be excessive.

Most people should be below 50 grams each day to attain ketosis. Consider that this won't give you numerous carb choices - except vegetables and smaller amounts of berries.

Summary

If you wish to enter ketosis and enjoy the entire metabolic great things about low carb diets, going below 50 grams of carbs each day could be necessary.

Eating too much Protein

Protein is an essential macronutrient that a lot of people don't get enough of. It could improve feelings of fullness and increase fat reduction better than other macronutrients. Generally speaking, considerably more protein should result in weight loss and improved body composition.

However, low carb dieters who eat a whole lot of lean animal foods can end up eating an excessive amount of it. When you take in extra protein that the body needs, a few of the proteins are converted into glucose through a process called *gluconeogenesis*. This can turn into a problem on very low-carb, ketogenic diets and stop the body from entering full-blown *ketosis*.

According to some scientists, a well-formulated low carb diet should be saturated in fat and moderate in protein. An excellent range to shoot for is 0.7-0.9 grams of protein per pound of body weight (1.5-2.0 grams per kg).

Summary

Excessive protein consumption on the low carb diet can prevent you from entering ketosis.

The fear of eating fat

A lot of people get nearly all their calories from dietary carbs - especially sugars and grains. If you remove this power source from your diet, you need to replace it with something else.

However, some people believe that eliminating fats over a low carb diet can make your daily diet even healthier. That is a huge mistake. Unless you eat carbs, you need to add fat to make up for it. Failing to do this may lead to hunger and malnutrition.

There is no scientific reason to fear fat - as long as you avoid trans fats and choose healthy ones like monounsaturated and omega-3 fats.

A fat intake of around 70% of total calories could be a great choice for a lot of low carb or ketogenic diets. To get fat in this range, you need to choose fatty cuts of meat and liberally add healthy fats to meals.

Summary

A very low carb diet should be saturated in fat. Otherwise, you will not get enough energy or nutrition to sustain yourself.

Not Replenishing Sodium

One of many mechanisms behind low carb diets is a decrease in insulin amounts. Insulin performs many functions inside you, such as telling fat cells to store up fat and your kidneys to retain sodium. Over a low carb diet, your insulin levels decrease and your body starts shedding excess sodium - and water along with it.

However, sodium is an essential electrolyte. Low sodium levels may become problematic whenever your kidneys excrete an excessive amount of it. That is one reason people get side effects on low carb diets, like *lightheadedness, fatigue, headaches, and constipation.*

The ultimate way to circumvent this problem is to add more sodium to your daily diet. You can do this by salting your foods - but if it doesn't suffice, try drinking a cup of broth each day.

Summary

Low carb diets lower insulin levels, making your kidneys excrete excess sodium. This may result in a mild sodium deficiency.

Quitting Too Early

Your body is made to preferentially burn carbs. Consequently, if carbs are always available, that's what the body uses for energy. If you drastically reduce on carbs, the body must shift to losing fat - which either originates from your daily diet or your body's stores. Normally it takes a couple of days for the body to adjust to burning primarily fat rather than carbs, where you will likely feel a little under the weather. That is called the *"keto flu"* and happens to many people that continue ultra-low carb diets.

If you feel sick after a few days, you might be tempted to stop your diet plan. However, remember that it might take 3-4 days for your body to adjust to your new regimen - with full adaptation taking several weeks. Therefore, it is critical to have patience initially and strictly stick to your diet.

Summary

On the low carb diet, normally it takes a couple of days to overcome unpleasant symptoms and many weeks for full adaptation. It's important to be patient and never abandon your daily diet too soon. Low carb diets may provide a potential cure for a few of the world's biggest health issues, including obesity and type 2 diabetes. This is good and is supported by science.

However, just reducing carbs is not enough to lose excess weight or boost health. Be sure to feed on a well-balanced diet and get enough exercise to accomplish optimal health.

Chapter 6

Ways to reduce your Carbohydrate Intake

Reducing carbohydrates can have major benefits for your well-being. Many studies show that low carb diets might help you lose weight and control diabetes or prediabetes. Listed below are easy methods to reduce your carb intake.

Eliminate Sugar-Sweetened Drinks

Sugar-sweetened beverages have become unhealthy. They're saturated in added sugar that is linked to a greater threat of insulin resistance, type 2 diabetes, and obesity when consumed excessively. A 12-ounce (354-ml) can of sugary soda contains 38 grams of carbs, and a 12-ounce sweetened iced tea has 36 grams of carbs. These come entirely from sugar. If you wish to eat fewer carbs, avoiding sugar-sweetened drinks should be among the first things you do.

If you wish to drink something refreshing having a taste, try adding some lime or lemon to club soda or iced tea. If needed, use a handful of low-calorie sweeteners.

Note:

Sweet drinks are saturated in carbs and added sugar. Avoiding them can significantly lessen your carbohydrate intake.

Cut back on Bread

Bread is often a staple food in lots of diets. Unfortunately, it is also quite saturated in carbs and generally lower in fiber. This is also true for white bread created from refined grains, which might negatively impact health insurance and weight. Actually, nutritious breads such as rye contain about 15 grams of carbs per slice. And a couple of these are dietary fiber, the only element of carbs that are not digested and absorbed.

Although wholegrain bread contains minerals and vitamins, a great many other foods are offering the same nutrients with much fewer carbs. These well-balanced meals have vegetables, nuts, and seeds. However, it could be tough to stop bread entirely. If you are finding it difficult, try among these delicious low carb bread recipes which are easy to create.

Note:

Whole-grain breads contain some crucial nutrients, but these are available in a great many other foods which can be reduced carbs.

Stop Drinking Juice

Unlike complete fruit, juice contains little to no fiber and is filled with sugar. Though it provides some minerals and vitamins, it's not much better than sugar-sweetened beverages with regards to sugar and carbs. That is true even for 100% juice. For example, 12oz (354 ml) of 100% apple juice contains 48 grams of carbs, most of its content is sugar.

You need to avoid juice completely. Instead, try flavoring your water with the addition of a slice of orange or lemon.

Note:

Juice contains as much carbs as sugar-sweetened beverages. Rather than drinking juice, put a little bit of fruit into water.

Choose Low carb Snacks

Carbs can truly add up quickly in snacks such as chips, pretzels, and crackers. These kinds of foods are also not so satisfying. One research found women felt fuller and ate 100 fewer calories at dinner if they ate a high-protein snack, in comparison to a low-protein one. Using a low carb snack that has protein may be the best strategy when hunger strikes between meals.

Here are some healthy snacks which contain significantly less than 5 grams of digestible (net) carbs per 1-oz (28-gram) serving and in addition some protein:

- **Almonds:** 6 grams of carbs, 3 of which are fiber.
- **Peanuts:** 6 grams of carbs, 2 of which are fiber.
- **Macadamia nut products:** 4 grams of carbs, 2 of which are fiber.
- **Hazelnuts:** 5 grams of carbs, 3 of which are fiber.
- **Pecans:** 4 grams of carbs, 3 of which are fiber.
- **Walnuts:** 4 grams of carbs, 2 of which are fiber.
- **Cheese:** Significantly less than 1 gram of carbs.

Note:

Be sure to possess healthy low carb snacks such as nuts and cheese readily available in the event you obtain hungry between meals.

Eat Eggs or Additional Low carb Breakfast Foods

Even smaller amounts of some breakfast foods tend to be saturated in carbs.

For example, one half-cup (55 grams) of granola cereal typically has around 30 grams of digestible carbs, even before adding milk.

Conversely, eggs are a perfect breakfast if you are trying to lessen carbs. To begin with, each egg contains significantly less than 1 gram of carbs. They're also an excellent way to obtain high-quality protein, that may help you experience full all night and eat fewer calories through the remaining daytime.

Also, eggs are versatile and may be prepared in lots of ways, including hard-boiling for an on-the-go breakfast.

For breakfast recipes featuring eggs along with other low carb foods, read this: 18 Low carb Breakfast Recipes.

Note

Choosing eggs or additional high-protein, low carb foods for breakfast might help you are feeling full and satisfied for several hours.

Use These Sweeteners instead of Sugar

Using sugar to sweeten foods and beverages is not a healthy performance, particularly on the low carb diet. One tablespoon of white or brown sugar has 12 grams of carbs using sucrose which is 50% fructose and 50% glucose.

Although honey might seem healthier, it's even higher in carbs. One tablespoon provides 17 grams of carbs, with roughly the same percentage of fructose and glucose as sugar. Learning to benefit from the natural flavor of foods without adding any sweetener may ultimately be best.

However, here are some safe sugar-free sweeteners that could even involve some modest health advantages:

Stevia: Stevia originates from the stevia plant, which started in South USA. In animal studies, it's been shown to support lower blood sugar and increase insulin sensitivity.

Erythritol: Erythritol is a kind of sugar alcohol that tastes like sugar, will not raise blood sugar levels or insulin amounts, and may assist in preventing cavities by killing plaque-causing bacteria.

Xylitol: Another sugar alcohol, xylitol also helps fight the bacteria that cause tooth decay. Furthermore, animal research suggests it could reduce insulin resistance and drive back obesity.

Note:

Using low-calorie sugar alternatives might help you retain your carb intake low without quitting sweetness altogether.

Ask for Veggies instead of Potatoes or Breads at Restaurants

Eating out could be challenging through the initial stages of the low carb diet. Even though you order meat or fish without breading or gravy, you'll typically get starch privately. This is *potatoes, pasta, bread or rolls*.

However, these starches can add 30 grams of carbs to your meal or even more. It depends on the portion size which is often quite large.

Instead, ask your server to substitute low carb vegetables instead of the high-carb foods. In case your meal already carries a side of vegetables, you could have another serving, so long as the vegetables are the non-starchy type.

Note

Getting vegetables rather than *potatoes, pasta, or bread* when eating dinner out can save many carbs.

Substitute Low carb Flours for Wheat Flour

Wheat flour is a high-carb ingredient generally in most baked goods, including breads, muffins, and cookies. It is also used for coating meat and fish ahead of sauteing or baking. Even whole wheat grains, which contain even more fiber than processed white flour, offer 61 grams of digestible carbs per 100 grams (3.5 ounces).

Fortunately, flours created from nut products and coconuts certainly are a great alternative and accessible at food markets and from trusted online retailers. 100 grams of almond flour contains significantly less than 11 grams of digestible carbs, and 100 grams of coconut flour contains 21 grams of digestible carbs.

These flours may be used to coat foods for sauteing, as well as with recipes that demand wheat flour. However, because they don't contain gluten, the texture of the finished product often will not be the same.

Almond and coconut flour tend to work best in recipes for muffins, pancakes, and similar soft, baked goods.

Note

Use almond or coconut flour instead of wheat flour in baked goods or when coating food ahead of sauteing or baking.

Replace Milk with Almond or Coconut Milk

Milk is nutritious, but it is also fairly saturated in carbs since it contains a kind of sugar called lactose. An 8-ounce (240 ml) glass of full-fat or low-fat milk contains 12-13 grams of carbs.

Adding a splash of milk to your tea or coffee is fine. But if you drink milk from the glassful or in lattes or shakes, you could find yourself contributing a whole lot of carbs.

There are many milk substitutes available. Typically, the most popular are coconut and almond milk, but there are also types created from various other nut products and hemp. Vitamin D, calcium, as well as other minerals and vitamins, are often put to improve vitamins and minerals. These drinks are mainly water, as well as the carb content material is usually surprisingly low. Most have 2 grams of digestible carbs or less per portion.

However, some contain sugar, so make sure to check the ingredient list and nutrition label to be sure you are getting an unsweetened, low carb beverage.

Note

Employ almond milk, coconut milk, or other alternative low carb milk substitutes instead of regular milk.

Emphasize Non-Starchy Veggies

Vegetables certainly are a valuable way to obtain nutrients and fiber over a low carb diet. In addition, they contain phytochemicals (plant compounds), a lot of which work as antioxidants that help protect you from diseases.

However, it is critical to select non-starchy types to keep your carb intake down. Vegetables and legumes, such as *carrots, beets, sweet potatoes, peas, lima beans, and corn,* are moderately saturated in carbs.

Fortunately, there are numerous delicious, nourishing low carb veggies you can eat.

Note

Select non-starchy vegetables to keep your carb intake low while maintaining a higher intake of nutrients and fiber.

Choose Dairy That's Low in Carbs

Milk products are delicious and are very healthy. To begin with, they contain calcium, magnesium along with other important minerals. Dairy also has *conjugated linoleic acid (CLA)*, a kind of fatty acid which has been shown to market fat loss in some studies.

However, some dairy foods are bad choices on the low carb diet. For example, fruit-flavored yogurt, frozen yogurt, and pudding tend to be packed with sugar and incredibly saturated in carbs.

Alternatively, *Greek yogurt and cheese* are lower in carbs and also have been shown to lessen appetite, promote fullness, improve body composition and reduce cardiovascular disease risk factors.

Here are some very good dairy choices, along with carb counts per 100 grams (3.5 oz):

- Simple Greek yogurt: 4 grams of carbs.
- Cheese (brie, mozzarella, cheddar, etc.): 1 gram of carbs.
- Ricotta cheese: 3 grams of carbs.
- Cottage cheese: 3 grams of carbs.

Note

Choose Greek yogurt and cheese to be able to maximize the benefits of dairy without carbs.

Eat Healthy High-Protein Foods

Eating an excellent protein source at every meal makes it easier to reduce on carbs, and it's particularly important if you are attempting to lose weight. Protein triggers the discharge in the *"fullness hormone" PYY*, reduces hunger, helps fight food cravings, and protects muscle tissue during weight loss.

Protein also offers a higher thermic value in comparison to fat or carbs, meaning your metabolic process increases more when digesting and metabolizing it.

<u>Be sure to has at least one serving out of this set of high-protein, low carb foods at each meal:</u>

- Meat
- Poultry
- Fish
- Eggs
- Nuts
- Cheese
- Cottage cheese
- Greek yogurt
- Whey protein powder.

Note:

Consuming protein at every meal might help you are feeling full, fight cravings and increase your metabolic rate.

Prepare Foods with Healthy Fats

Fat replaces some carbs and typically accounts for over 50% of calories over a low carb diet. Therefore, it is important to choose fats that not merely add flavor but also benefit your wellbeing.

Two of the healthiest choices are *virgin coconut oil and extra-virgin olive oil. Virgin coconut oil* is an extremely saturated fat that's very stable at high cooking temperatures. The majority of its fat is *medium-chain triglycerides (MCTs)*, which might reduce stomach fat and increase **HDL** cholesterol.

Also, these MCTs could decrease appetite. In a single report, men who ate an MCT-rich breakfast ate significantly fewer calories at lunch than men who ate a breakfast saturated in long-chain triglycerides.

Extra-virgin olive oil has been shown to lessen blood pressure, enhance the function of the cells lining your arteries and assist in preventing putting on weight.

Note:

Preparing low carb foods with healthy fats can boost flavor, promote feelings of fullness and improve your wellbeing.

Reading Food Labels

Taking a look at food labels can offer valuable information regarding the carb content of packaged foods. The main element is knowing where you can appear and whether any calculations have to be done.

If you live outside the US, the dietary fiber in the carbs section might be recently reduced. If you reside in the US, you can deduct the grams of fibers from your carbs to obtain the digestible ("net") carb content. You'll want to take a look at how many portions are contained in the package, as it's several.

In case a trail mix contains 7 grams of carbs per portion and a complete of 4 servings, you'll turn out eating 28 grams of carbs if you eat the complete bag.

Note:

Reading food labels might help you regulate how many carbs are in packaged foods.

Count Carbs Having a Nutrition Tracker

A nutrition tracker is an excellent tool for monitoring your daily diet. Most are obtainable as apps for smartphones and tablets, as well as online.

Whenever you enter your meal intake for every meal and snack, carbs, as well as other nutrients, are automatically calculated.

A few of the most popular nourishment tracking programs are *My Fitness Pal, Spark People, Fit Day, and Cron-o-Meter.*

These programs calculate your nutrient needs based on your body weight, age along with other factors, nevertheless, you can customize your daily carb goal and change it out when you like.

A lot of the info in the meals databases is trustworthy. However, take into account that a few of these programs allow visitors to bring custom nutrition information that might not continually be accurate.

Note:

Using a nutrition tracking app or online program might help you monitor and fine-tune your carb intake.

Transitioning to a healthy low carb lifestyle could be relatively easy when you have the proper information and tools.

Chapter 7

Junk Foods You Can Eat on the Low Carb Diet

Sticking with a low carb diet when eating out could be hard, especially at fast-food restaurants. That's because these meals tend to be based on breads, tortillas, along with other high-carb items. Nonetheless, most fast-food restaurants offer the right low carb options, and several items can simply be modified to suit your lifestyle.

Listed below are delicious junk foods you can eat over a low carb diet.

Sub in a tub

Submarine sandwiches have become saturated in carbs. An average sub has at least 50 grams of carbs, the majority of which come from your bun. Ordering your sub "in a tub" (in a bowl or container), instead of on the bun, can help you save more than 40 grams of carbs.

The carb counts for sub-in-a-tub options may appear something similar to this:

- *Turkey breast and provolone*: 8 grams of carbs, 1 of which is fiber.

- *Club supreme*: 11 grams of carbs, 2 of which are fiber.
- *Chicken salad*: 9 grams of carbs, 3 of which are fiber.
- *California club*: 9 grams of carbs, 4 which are fiber.

Although the word "sub in a tub" originated at Jersey Mike's, you can order your meal in this manner from any sub sandwich shop, including Subway.

Summary

To reduce carbs while keeping protein intake high, order your preferred sub sandwich "in a tub" or a salad.

KFC Grilled Chicken

Fried chicken is not a healthy choice. To begin with, the chicken absorbs a lot of oil during frying. Heating vegetable oils to high temperatures produce harmful compounds that could boost your risk of cardiovascular disease, cancer, as well as other health issues.

Furthermore, fried chicken contains about 8-11 grams of carbs per medium-size piece. Grilled chicken is usually a

119

greater option and is offered by many Kentucky Fried Chicken (**KFC**) franchises. Each little bit of grilled KFC chicken has significantly less than 1 gram of carbs.

For side dishes, green beans contain 2 grams of digestible carbs per portion and are undoubtedly your best option. Coleslaw is next, at 10 grams of digestible carbs.

Summary

Choose 3 bits of grilled chicken having a side of green beans for any balanced meal which has less than 10 grams of carbs.

Tea or coffee with cream

Coffee and tea are carb-free beverages. They're also saturated in caffeine, which gives some impressive benefits. Caffeine may increase your mood, metabolic process, and mental and physical performance.

If you want milk in your cup of joe, coffee houses and fast-food eateries often offer half-and-half. A single-serving container has about 0.5 grams of carbs. Heavy cream's almost carb-free and sometimes obtainable.

However, it has about 50 calories per tablespoon (15 ml), in comparison to 20 calories for half-and-half.

Some coffee houses also offer soy or almond milk. Unsweetened versions of the milk substitutes provide minimal carbs per 2-tablespoon (30 ml) serving.

Summary

If you like to drink coffee with milk or cream, require half-and-half, heavy cream, or unsweetened soy or almond milk.

Chipotle salad or bowl

Chipotle is a Mexican fast-food restaurant that has been extremely popular. Many people contemplate it as healthier than other chains since it uses high-quality ingredients and emphasizes animal welfare and sustainable farming practices. Chipotle also helps it be very easy to produce low carb meals. A salad with meat or chicken, grilled vegetables, and guacamole contains 14 grams of total carbs, 8 of which are fiber.

This meal also provides about 30 grams of high-quality protein. A higher protein and fiber intake can boost your production from the gut hormones peptide YY (PYY) and cholecystokinin (CCK), which tell the human brain you're full and assist in preventing overeating.

Though vinaigrette can be obtained, generous servings of guacamole and salsa make salad dressing unnecessary.

Additionally, Chipotle has a helpful online nutrition calculator which allows you to start to see the exact carb content of the meal.

Summary

Decide on a salad with meat, vegetables, salsa, and guacamole to get a satisfying meal with 6 grams of digestible carbs.

Lettuce-wrapped burger

A bunless burger wrapped in lettuce is a typical low-carb, fast-food meal. It's saturated in protein, essentially carb-free, and offered by all fast-food burger establishments. You can further customize your burger with the addition of the following low carb toppings or additions, based on availability and personal preferences:

- *Cheese*: Significantly less than 1 gram of carbs per slice

- *Bacon*: Significantly less than 1 gram of carbs per slice

- *Mustard*: Significantly less than 1 gram of carbs per tablespoon
- *Mayo*: Significantly less than 1 gram of carbs per tablespoon
- *Onions*: 1 gram of digestible carbs per slice
- *Tomato*: Significantly less than 1 gram of digestible carbs per slice
- *Guacamole*: 3 grams of digestible carbs per 1/4 cup (60 grams)

Summary

Top your bunless burger with condiments and further toppings to has flavor while minimizing carb intake.

Panera Breads power breakfast bowl

Panera Bread is a café-style restaurant featuring sandwiches, pastries, soups, salads, and coffee. A lot of the breakfast items are saturated in carbs. However, two selections using their menu work well for the low carb breakfast.

The Energy Breakfast Egg Bowl with Steak features steak, tomatoes, avocado, and 2 eggs. It offers 5 grams of carbs and 20 grams of protein.

The Energy Breakfast Egg White Bowl with Turkey contains egg whites, spinach, bell peppers, and basil for 7 grams of carbs and 25 grams of protein. Starting your day with a high-protein breakfast promotes feelings of fullness and decreases appetite by reducing degrees of the hunger hormone ghrelin.

Summary

Choose an egg-based breakfast with meat and vegetables at Panera Loaf of bread to maintain carb intake low and control hunger levels.

Buffalo wings

Buffalo wings are delicious and fun to eat. They could also be considered a low carb option at pizza places and sports bars, based on how they're prepared. Traditionally, buffalo wings are covered in a spicy red sauce created from vinegar and hot red peppers.

An order of the buffalo wings typically has 0-3 grams of carbs per portion. By contrast, various other sauces can add a significant quantity of carbs, especially sweet types, such as barbecue, teriyaki, and anything made from honey.

Sometimes the wings are breaded or battered and fried, which is particularly common for boneless wings. Therefore, ensure to ask the way the wings are created and order yours without breading or batter. Buffalo wings will also be usually served with carrots, celery, and ranch dressing.

Although they're higher in carbs than a great many other vegetables, carrots are fine to eat in small quantities. A half-cup (60 grams) of carrot strips contains about 5 grams of net carbs.

Summary

Choose non-breaded buffalo wings with traditional sauce, celery, and some carrot strips to make a meal with under 10 grams of net carbs.

Bacon or Sause and Eggs

Sometimes the easiest breakfast option could be the most delicious, such as bacon or sause and eggs. This traditional breakfast combination offered by most fast-food restaurants has minimal carbs. Also, eggs might help hold you full and satisfied all night.

In one report on overweight young women, eating sause and eggs for breakfast helped reduce appetite. In addition, it lowered blood sugar levels and insulin while reducing calorie consumption at lunch, in comparison to a low-protein, higher-carb breakfast. However, cured bacon and sauses are processed meat products, which were linked to an increased risk of cardiovascular disease and cancer. Because of this, most medical researchers advise against a higher intake of foods.

Summary

Bacon or sause with eggs provides hardly any carbs, reduces hunger, and can help you look full all night. However, limit your intake of processed meats, as they're associated with an increased threat of cardiovascular disease and cancer.

Arby's sandwich with no bun or bread

Arby's is among the largest fast-food sandwich chains in America. Although Roast Beef Classic is its original &

most popular item, Arby's has many other options, including brisket, steak, ham, chicken, and turkey.

These could be ordered minus the bread for a very tasty low-carb, high-protein meal. The business website offers a nutrition calculator, and that means you can customize your order to keep carbs in your target range. For example, you may select Smokehouse Brisket with Gouda cheese, sauce, and a side salad for 5 grams of digestible carbs and 32 grams of protein.

Summary

Use Arby's diet calculator to create a high-protein meal in your target carb range.

Antipasto salad

Fast-food Italian restaurants are most widely known for high-carb foods like pizza, pasta, and subs. *Antipasto salad* offers a delicious, low carb alternative.

This salad is traditionally served as an appetizer, comprising assorted meats, cheese, olives, and vegetables topped with an olive oil-based dressing. However, it could be ordered in a more substantial portion as an entrée.

An entrée-size serving of antipasto salad is abundant with protein and has less than 10 grams of digestible carbs.

Summary

Choose antipasto salad for just a filling, low carb meal at an Italian fast-food restaurant.

Subway double chicken chopped salad

Subway may be the most popular fast-food sandwich shop worldwide. Lately, the chain continues to be offering chopped salads that may be customized with protein and vegetables of your decision. Probably one of the most satisfying and nutritious choices may be the *Double Chicken Chopped Salad* with Avocado. It has 10 grams of total carbs, 4 of which are fiber, and also a whopping 36 grams of protein.

Avocados are abundant with heart-healthy monounsaturated fat and fiber. Eating them at lunch could even result in lower calorie consumption at the next meal.

A summary of Subway salads, along with complete nutrition information, are available here.

Summary

Order a salad with double meat, vegetables, and avocados for your delicious and satisfying Subway meal.

Burrito bowl

Many people regard burritos as a favorite food. They typically contain meat, vegetables, rice, and beans wrapped in a big flour tortilla. This leads to a meal that may easily pack a lot more than 100 grams of carbs. However, almost every Mexican restaurant gives you to omit the tortilla along with other high-carb items.

This is referred to as a *burrito bowl* or *"bare" burrito.*

A burrito bowl made out of meat, grilled onions, bell peppers, and salsa can be a delicious and satisfying meal that delivers significantly less than 10 grams of digestible carbs.

Summary

Select a burrito bowl or "bare" burrito for the fantastic flavor of a normal burrito with hardly any carbs.

McDonald's breakfast sandwich with no bread

McDonald's may be the most popular fast-food chain on the planet, with an increase of more than 36,000 restaurants worldwide by 2018. Though it is best known for burgers just like the Big Mac and Quarter Pounder, its Egg McMuffin and Sause McMuffin breakfast sandwiches may also be very popular.

These breakfast entrées contain an English muffin with one egg, a slice of American cheese, and ham or sause.

Each sandwich contains 29 grams of carbs. However, ordering either of the items minus the muffin will certainly reduce the carb content material to 2 grams or less.

It's also smart to order 2 low carb sandwiches, as each one is only going to provide about 12 grams of protein.

Summary

At McDonald's, order 2 eggs or Sause McMuffins with no bread for any satisfying meal with 4 grams or less of carbs and 24 grams of protein.

Arby's roast turkey farmhouse salad

As mentioned above, ordering a bun-less Arby's sandwich is a superb low carb option. Additionally, Arby's offers a Roast Turkey Farmhouse Salad featuring roast turkey, bacon, cheese, mixed greens, and tomatoes. It contains simply 8 grams of carbs, 2 of which are fiber, along with 22 grams of protein. Just ensure never to confuse it using the Crispy Chicken Farmhouse Salad, which has chicken that has been breaded and fried. It packs 26 grams of total carbs.

Summary

Choose Arby's Roast Turkey Farmhouse Salad for an excellent mix of flavors and textures with 6 grams of digestible carbs. Even though you just see high-carb items on a menu, a delicious low carb meal could be created for the most part fast-food restaurants by causing simple substitutions. Although junk food is unquestionably much less healthy than the meals you could prepare at home, it's sound to know what things to order if it is your only choice.

Chapter 8

Foods to avoid (or Limit) on the Low Carb Diet

A low carb diet might help you lose weight and control diabetes along with other circumstances. Some high-carb foods have to be avoided, such as sugar-sweetened drinks, cake, and candy.

Yet, determining which staple foods to limit is more difficult. A few of these foods are even relatively healthy - just unsuitable for any low carb diet because of a lot of carbs. Your total daily carb target determines whether you will need to limit a few of these foods or prevent them altogether. Low carb diets typically contain 20-150 grams of carbs each day, Based on personal tolerance.

Listed below are foods to avoid or limit over a low carb diet.

Bread and grains

Bread is a staple food in lots of cultures. It will come in assorted forms, including loaves, rolls, bagels, and flatbreads, such as tortillas. However, many of these are saturated in carbs. That is true for whole-grain varieties as well as those created from refined flour.

Although carb counts vary based on ingredients and food portion sizes, here are the common counts for popular breads.

- *White bread (1 slice):* 14 grams of carbs, 1 which is fiber
- Whole-wheat breads (1 slice): 17 grams of carbs, 2 which are fiber
- *Flour tortilla (10-inch):* 36 grams of carbs, 2 of which are fiber
- *Bagel (3-inch):* 29 grams of carbs, 1 which is fiber

Depending on your carb tolerance, eating a sandwich, burrito, or bagel could put you near or higher your daily limit.

If you even now want to take pleasure from bread, help to make your own low carb loaves at the home.

Most grains, including rice, wheat, and oats, will also be saturated in carbs and have to be limited or avoided on the low carb diet.

Summary

Most breads and grains, including whole grains and whole-grain loafs of bread, are too much in carbs to add to a low carb diet.

Some fruit

A higher intake of fruits & vegetables has consistently been associated with a lower threat of cancer and cardiovascular disease.

However, many fruits are saturated in carbs and could not be ideal for low carb diets. An average serving of fruit is 1 cup (120 grams) or 1 small piece. For example, a little apple contains 21 grams of carbs, 4 of which come from fiber. On the very-low carb diet, it's probably smart to avoid some fruits, especially sweet and dried fruits, that have high carb counts:

- *Banana (1 medium):* 27 grams of carbs, 3 of which are fiber
- *Raisins (1 ounce / 28 grams):* 22 grams of carbs, 1 which is fiber
- *Dates (2 large):* 36 grams of carbs, 4 which are fiber

Mango, sliced (1 cup / 165 grams): 28 grams of carbs, 3 of which are fiber Berries are lower in sugar and higher in fiber than other fruits.

Consequently, smaller amounts - around 1/2 cup (50 grams) - could be enjoyed even on very-low carb diets.

Summary

Many fruits should be limited on the low carb diet, based on your carb tolerance. Having said that, berries can often be enjoyed.

Starchy vegetables

Most diets allow an unlimited intake of low-starch vegetables. Many vegetables have become saturated in fiber, which may aid weight loss and blood sugar level control.

However, some high-starch vegetables contain much more digestible carbs than dietary fiber and really should be limited to a low carb diet.

What's more, if you are carrying out a very low carb diet, your best choice is to order to avoid these starchy vegetables completely.

- *Corn (1 cup / 175 grams):* 41 grams of carbs, 5 of which are fiber
- *Potato (1 medium):* 37 grams of carbs, 4 of which are fiber
- *Sweet Potato/yam (1 medium):* 24 grams of carbs, 4 which are fiber
- *Beets, cooked (1 cup / 150 grams):* 16 grams of carbs, 4 which are fiber

Notably, you can enjoy several low carb vegetables on a low carb diet.

Summary

Although some vegetables are lower in carbs, several are very high. You need to select mostly non-starchy, high-fiber vegetables when limiting your carb intake.

Pasta

Pasta is a versatile and inexpensive staple but high in carbs. One cup (250 grams) of cooked pasta contains 43 grams of carbs, only 3 of which are fiber. The same amount of whole-wheat pasta is a slightly better option at 37 grams of carbs, including 6 grams of fiber. Over a low carb diet, eating spaghetti or other styles of pasta is not a good idea if you don't eat an extremely small portion, which isn't realistic for many people.

If you are craving pasta but don't want to debate your carb limit, try making spiralized vegetables or shirataki noodles instead.

Summary

Both standard and whole-wheat pasta are saturated in carbs. Spiralized vegetables or shirataki noodles offer healthy low carb alternatives.

Cereal

It's popular that sugary breakfast cereals have a large number of carbs. However, you might be surprised by the carb matters of healthy cereals.

For example, 1 cup (90 grams) of cooked regular or instant oatmeal provides 32 grams of carbs, only 4 of which are fiber.

Steel-cut oats are less processed than other styles of oatmeal and are generally considered healthier.

However, only 1/2 cup (45 grams) of cooked steel-cut oats has 29 grams of carbs, including 5 grams of fiber. Whole-grain cereals tend to pack a lot more. A 1/2 cup

(61 grams) of granola harbors 37 grams of carbs and 7 grams of fiber, as the same amount of Grape Nuts has an impressive 46 grams of carbs with 5 grams of fiber.

Depending on your individual carb goal, a plate of cereal could easily put you over your total carb limit - even before milk is added.

Summary

Healthy, whole-grain cereals are saturated in carbs and really should exist prevented or minimized over a low carb diet.

Beer

Alcohol could be enjoyed in moderation on the low carb diet. Dry wine hardly contains any carbs and hard liquor. However, beer is rather saturated in carbs. A 12-ounce (356-ml) can of beer packs 13 grams of carbs, normally. Also, light beer contains 6 grams per can. Also, studies claim that liquid carbs tend to promote putting on weight a lot more than carbs from solid food.

That's because liquid carbs aren't as filling as solid food and do not appear to diminish your appetite nearly just as much.

Summary

Avoid drinking beer over a low carb diet. Dry wine and spirits are better alcohol options.

Sweetened Yogurt

Yogurt is tasty, versatile food. Although natural yogurt is fairly lower in carbs, many people tend to eat fruit-flavored, sweetened low-fat, or non-fat yogurt. Sweetened yogurt often contains as many carbs as a dessert. One cup (245 grams) of non-fat sweetened fruit yogurt can have as much as 47 grams of carbs, which is even greater than a comparable serving of ice cream.

However, selecting a 1/2 cup (123 grams) of plain Greek yogurt topped with 1/2 cup (50 grams) of blackberries or raspberries could keep digestible carbs under 10 grams.

Summary

Sweetened low-fat or non-fat yogurt often offers as many carbs as ice cream as well as other desserts.

Juice

Juice is among the worst drinks you may drink on a low carb diet. Though it provides some nutrients, juice is extremely saturated in fast-digesting carbs that cause your blood glucose to improve rapidly.

For example, 12 ounces (355 ml) of apple juice harbors 48 grams of carbs. That is a lot more than soda, which has 39 grams. Grape juice offers a whopping 60 grams of carbs per 12-ounce (355-ml) serving.

Although vegetable juice doesn't contain nearly as many carbs as its fruit counterparts, a 12-ounce (355-ml) serving still has 16 grams of carbs, only 2 of which result from fiber.

Also, juice is another example of liquid carbs that your brain's appetite center might not process just as solid carbs. Drinking juice can result in increased hunger and diet later in your day.

Summary

Fruit juice can be a high-carb beverage that needs to be limited or avoided, especially over a low carb diet.

Low-fat and fat-free salad dressings

A multitude of salads could be enjoyed regularly on the low carb diet. However, commercial dressings - especially low-fat and fat-free varieties - often find yourself adding more carbs than you may expect. For instance, 2 tablespoons (30 ml) of fat-free French dressing contain 10 grams of carbs. The same part of fat-free ranch dressing has 11 grams of carbs.

Many people commonly use more than 2 tablespoons (30 ml), particularly on a big entrée salad. To reduce carbs, dress your salad having a creamy, full-fat dressing. Better yet, make use of a splash of vinegar and olive oil, which is associated with improved heart health insurance and may aid fat loss.

Summary

Avoid fat-free and low-fat salad dressings, which are usually saturated in carbs. Use creamy dressings or olive oil and vinegar instead.

Beans and Legumes

Beans and legumes are nutritious foods. They can provide many health advantages, including reduced inflammation and cardiovascular disease risk.

Although saturated in fiber, in addition, they have a fair amount of carbs. Based on personal tolerance, you might be able to consist of small amounts over a low carb diet.

Listed below are the carb counts for 1 cup (160-200 grams) of cooked beans and legumes:

- *Lentils:* 40 grams of carbs, 16 of which are fiber
- *Peas:* 25 grams of carbs, 9 of which are fiber
- *Black beans:* 41 grams of carbs, 15 of which are fiber
- *Pinto beans:* 45 grams of carbs, 15 of which are fiber
- *Chickpeas:* 45 grams of carbs, 12 of which are fiber
- *Kidney beans:* 40 grams of carbs, 13 of which are fiber

Summary

Beans and legumes are healthy, high fiber foodstuffs. You can small amounts on the low carb diet, based on your day-by-day carb limit.

Honey or Sugar in any form

You're probably well aware that foods saturated in sugar, such as cookies, chocolate, and cake, are off-limits over a low carb diet.

However, may very well not recognize that natural types of sugar can possess as many carbs as white sugar. Most of them are even higher in carbs when measured in tablespoons.

Listed below are the carb counts for just one tablespoon of various kinds of sugar:

- *White sugar:* 12.6 grams of carbs
- *Maple syrup:* 13 grams of carbs
- *Agave nectar:* 16 grams of carbs
- *Honey:* 17 grams of carbs

Also, these sweeteners provide little to no vitamins and minerals. When carb consumption is bound, you must prefer nutritious, high-fiber carb sources.

To sweeten foods or beverages without adding carbs, select a healthy sweetener instead.

Summary

If you're on a low carb diet, avoid sugar, honey, maple syrup, and other styles of sugar, that are saturated in carbs but lower in nutrients.

Chips and Crackers

Chips and crackers are popular snacks, but their carbs can add up quickly. One ounce (28 grams) of tortilla chips contains 18 grams of carbs, only one 1 which is fiber. That is about 10-15 average-sized chips.

Crackers vary in carb content based on processing. However, even whole-wheat crackers contain about 19 grams of carbs per 1 ounce (28 grams), including 3 grams of fiber (55). Processed snacks are usually consumed in large quantities in a brief period of time. You need to avoid them, particularly if you're over a carb-restricted diet.

Summary

Avoid eating chips, and crackers, along with other refined, grain-based snacks while on a low carb diet.

Milk

Milk is a superb way to obtain several nutrients, including calcium, potassium, and many B vitamins. However, it is also fairly saturated in carbs. Dairy supplies the same 12-13 grams of carbs per 8 ounces (240 ml) as low-fat and fat-free varieties.

If you are only using a tablespoon or two (15-30 ml) in coffee once a day you might be in a position to include smaller amounts of milk in your low carb diet.

However, cream or half-and-half are better options if you eat coffee more often since these contain minimal carbs.

If you enjoy drinking milk from the glass or use it to create lattés or smoothies, consider trying unsweetened almond or coconut milk instead.

Summary

Adding a handful of milk to coffee once a day is unlikely to cause problems on the low carb diet. Do not drink it in large quantities.

Gluten-free Cooked Food

Gluten is often a protein in wheat, barley, and rye. Gluten-free diets have grown to be very popular lately and are necessary for people who have celiac disease. Celiac disease can be an autoimmune condition where your gut becomes inflamed in response to gluten. Having said that, gluten-free breads, muffins, as well as other baked goods aren't typically lower in carbs. They often boast a lot more carbs than their glutenous counterparts.

Also, the flour used to create these foods is normally created from starches and grains that tend to raise glucose levels rapidly.

Sticking to entire foods or using almond or coconut flour to create your low carb baked goods is an improved strategy than eating processed gluten-free foods.

Summary

Gluten-free breads and muffins are often as saturated in carbs as traditional baked goods. They're also often made out of carb sources that raise blood sugar levels quickly.

Bottom line

When carrying out a low carb diet, it is critical to choose foods that are highly nutritious but lower in carbs. Some foods should be minimized while some avoided altogether. Your alternatives depend partly on your personal carb tolerance. For the time being, concentrate on eating many healthy foods.

Chapter 9

Reasons You are not Losing Weight on the Low carb Diet

Low carb diets are amazing. That is a scientific fact. However, much like any diet, people sometimes stop losing before they reach their desired weight.

Here are the best 15 explanations why you're not slimming down over a low carb diet.

You Are Losing Weight, You Just Don't Understand It

Weight loss is not a linear process. If you weigh yourself each day, you will see days once the scale falls along with other days when it rises. It doesn't imply that the dietary plan isn't working, as long as the overall trend is going downwards.

Many people lose a whole lot of weight in the first week on the low carb diet; nonetheless, it is mainly water weight. Weight loss will decelerate significantly following this initial phase. Of course, slimming down is not like losing fat.

It's possible, particularly if you're not used to strength training, that you are gaining muscle at the same time as you're losing weight.

To ensure that you're losing, use something apart from just the level. Make use of a measuring tape to measure your waist and also have the body fat measured monthly or so. Also, take pictures. Observe how your clothes fit. If you are looking thinner and your clothes are looser, you are losing weight no matter what the size says.

Summary

Fat loss isn't linear, and there's far more to weight than simply body fat. Exercise patience and use different ways of measuring than the scale.

You're not reducing on Carbohydrates Enough

Some people tend to be more carb sensitive than others. If you're feeding on low carb and your weight starts to plateau, you might reduce on carbs even more. If so, go under 50 grams of carbs each day. When you are under 50 grams each day, you are going to need to eliminate most fruits from your diet, although you could have berries in smaller amounts.

If it doesn't work either, going under 20 grams temporarily could work. You then are eating just protein, healthy fats, and leafy vegetables.

To ensure that you're eating low-carb, use a free online nutrition tracker and log your meal intake for some time.

Summary

If you're carb sensitive, you might temporarily eliminate all high-carb foods and eat much less than 50 grams of carbs each day.

You're Stressed Regularly

Unfortunately, it is not enough to just eat healthily and exercise. You need to ensure that the body is functioning optimally and your hormonal environment is favorable. Being stressed regularly keeps your body in a consistent state of "fight or flight" - with elevated degrees of stress hormones like cortisol.

Having chronically elevated cortisol levels can boost your hunger and cravings for processed foods. If you wish to reduce stress, try meditation and yoga breathing exercises. Reduce on distractions like online news, and reading new books instead.

Summary

Chronic stress can have side effects on your hormonal environment, making you hungrier and preventing you from slimming down.

You're Not Consuming Real Food

A low carb diet is approximately more than simply cutting your intake of carbs. You must replace those carbohydrates with real, nutritious foods. Dispose all processed low carb products like Atkins bars, because they are not real food rather than good for your wellbeing. Stick to meat, fish, eggs, vegetables and healthy fats if you want to lose weight. Also, *"treats"* like paleo cookies and brownies could cause problems despite that they're made out of healthy ingredients. They must be considered occasional treats, not something you eat every day.

Additionally, it is vital that you eat enough fat. If you try to reduce carbs and fat at exactly the same time, you'll be ravenously hungry and feel bad. Eating a diet plan with only protein is an extremely bad idea. Low-carb, high-fat and modest protein may be the strategy to use if you wish to enter *ketosis*, which may be the optimal hormonal environment to burn surplus fat.

Summary

You need to displace the carbs with real, nutritious foods. To lose excess weight, stick to meat, fish, eggs, healthy fats and vegetables.

You're Eating Too Many Nuts

Nut products are real foods, without doubt about that. Also, they are high in fat. For instance, about 70% from the calories in almonds result from fat. However, nuts are simple to overeat. Their crunchiness and high energy density provide you with the ability to eat huge amounts of these without feeling full.

Personally, I can eat a bag of nuts but still not feel satisfied, despite the fact that the bag contains more calories when compared to a meal. If you are snacking on nut products each day (or worse, nut butters), it's likely that you're just taking in so many calories.

Summary

Nuts use a high energy denseness and are an easy task to overeat. If you are constantly snacking on nuts, try eliminating them.

You are not Sleeping Enough

Rest is incredibly very important to general health, and studies also show that the insomnia correlates with putting on weight and obesity. Too little sleep could make you feel hungrier. It will cause you to be tired and less motivated to exercise and eat healthy. Sleep is among the pillars of health. If you are doing everything right but nonetheless not getting proper rest, you won't start to see the results you may expect. When you have a sleeping disorder, see a medical expert. They are generally easily treatable.

Some ideas to improve sleep:

- Avoid caffeine after 2 pm
- Rest in complete darkness
- Avoid alcohol and physical activity in the last few hours before sleep
- Take action relaxing before slumber, like reading

- Try to go to sleep at the same time every night

Summary

Sleep is completely crucial for optimal wellbeing. Studies show insomnia can make you put on weight.

You're eating too much Dairy

Another low carb food that may cause problems for a lot of is dairy. Some milk products, despite being lower in carbs, remain pretty saturated in protein. Protein, like carbs, can boost insulin amounts, which drives energy into storage. The amino acid composition of dairy protein helps it be very potent at spiking insulin. Actually, dairy proteins can spike insulin just as much as white bread.

While you might seem to tolerate milk products merely fine, eating them often and spiking insulin could be detrimental to the metabolic adaptation that must occur to be able to reap the entire great things about low carb diets.

In cases like this, avoid milk and reduce the cheese, yogurt and cream. Butter is okay, as it is quite lower in protein and lactose and for that reason won't spike insulin.

Summary

The amino acid composition of dairy proteins makes them spike insulin fairly effectively. Try eating less dairy.

You're Not Exercising Right (or whatsoever)

You shouldn't exercise only to burn calories. The calories burned during exercise are often insignificant and may easily be negated by eating several extra bites of food at another meal. However, exercise is crucial for both physical and mental health. Exercise might help you lose weight by improving your metabolic health, upping your muscle tissue and causing you to feel awesome. But it is critical to do the proper sort of exercise. Only cardio around the treadmill machine is unlikely to offer great results and performing too much could even be detrimental.

Lifting weights: This can greatly increase your hormonal environment and boost your muscle mass, which can only help you lose weight over time.

Intensive training: Doing high-intensity intervals is a superb type of cardio that boosts your metabolism and raises your degrees of hgh.

Low intensity: Being active and doing some low-intensity work like walking is a superb idea. The body was made to maneuver around, not sit down in a chair all day long.

Summary

The right types of exercise transform your hormones, boost your muscle tissue and cause you to feel awesome.

You're Eating Too Many "Healthy" Sugars

If you're over a low carb or ketogenic diet, "healthy" sugars like coconut sugar or raw cane sugar are simply as bad as plain sugar. They are saturated in carbs and will completely stop your body from adapting to the dietary plan. This also pertains to honey, agave nectar and many others.

Zero-calorie sweeteners are fine for many people, but you may want to consider limiting them when you have trouble slimming down. In addition, they often contain digestible carbs as fillers.

Summary

Despite being natural, sweeteners like honey and raw cane sugar are simply as saturated in carbs as standard sugar.

You Might Have a Health Condition Making Things Difficult

Certain medications are known to stimulate putting on weight. If you go through the list of side effects of the drug you are taking and find *"putting on weight"* on the list, schedule an appointment with your doctor. Perhaps there is another drug available it that doesn't stimulate weight gain.

If you are doing everything ideal but still aren't getting good results, you might have an underlying medical problem. Many hormonal disorders could cause problems slimming down, particularly *hypothyroidism*.

If so, schedule an appointment with your doctor. Explain you are having problems slimming down and that you would like to eliminate any medical issues.

Summary

Particular medical issues and medications could cause weight problems. See a medical expert to discuss your alternatives.

You're Constantly Eating

It really is a persistent myth in health circles that everyone should be taking many, smaller meals during the day. It has actually been studied thoroughly. There is no advantage in eating more frequent and smaller sized meals. It is natural for humans to eat fewer meals each day and sometimes go long periods without food.

Some people take action called intermittent fasting, eating in an 8-hour window every day or doing 24-hour fasts 1-2 occasions per week. This is very beneficial to break via a plateau.

Summary

There is no proven benefit to eating many, smaller meals each day. Make an effort eating fewer meals and consider giving intermittent fasting a go.

You're Cheating too often

For those who have the ability to control themselves, having cheat meals or days once in a while could be fine. For others, especially those who find themselves susceptible to food addiction, having cheat meals will probably do more harm than good. If you are cheating often, either with "small cheats" occasionally or whole days where you take in nothing but processed foods, it can easily ruin your progress. Having more than 1-2 cheat meals weekly (or one cheat day) is likely to be excessive.

If you cannot control yourself around processed foods no matter how you try, you might have food addiction. If so, completely removing the junk food from your life is actually a good idea.

Summary

Some people can eat processed foods once in a while without ruining their progress, but it doesn't connect with everyone. For others, cheat meals can do more harm than great.

You're Ingesting too many Calories

By the end of your day, calories do matter. One of many factors low carb and ketogenic diets are so effective is that they reduce appetite and make people eat fewer overall calories without trying. If you are not slimming down but are doing all of the best things, try counting calories for some time.

Again, create a free of charge account with an internet nourishment tracker and track your intake for any few days. Go for a deficit of 500 calories each day, which theoretically should cause you to lose 1 pound of weight weekly (though it doesn't always work used).

Summary

You'll be able to eat a lot of calories which you stop slimming down. Make an effort counting calories and shoot for a deficit of 500 calories each day for some time.

You do not have Realistic Expectations

By the end of your day, weight loss takes time. It is a marathon - not really a sprint. Losing 1-2 pounds weekly is an authentic goal. Some people will lose weight faster than that, while some will lose weight even more slowly. But you'll want to take into account that not everyone can appear to be an exercise model. Sooner or later, you may reach a healthy set stage weight, which might be above everything you initially wished for.

Summary

It's important to set realistic expectations. Weight-loss takes a very long time, if not everyone would look like an exercise model.

You've Been "Cutting" for too much time

We don't think it's wise to maintain a calorie deficit for too much time at the same time. The leanest people on the planet (bodybuilders and fitness models) never do that. They are doing cycles of *"bulking"* and *"cutting."* If you eat at a calorie deficit for most months (or years), eventually your metabolic process may decelerate.

If you have been dieting for a long period, a two-month period where you try to *"maintain"* and gain a little bit of muscle could be what you should get things started again. Of course, this won't mean eating bad foods, just more of the nice stuff. After all of these months are over, you can start *"dieting"* again.

Chapter 10

How Much Carbs Should You Eat Per Day to Lose Excess Weight?

Low carb diets can be quite effective for weight loss, according to analysis. Reducing carbs will lessen your appetite and cause automatic weight loss, or fat loss with no need to depend calories. For most people, a minimal carb diet allows them to eat until fullness, feel satisfied, but still lose weight. The amount of carbs a person should eat each day for weight loss varies based on how old they are, sex, physique, and activity levels.

This chapter reviews how many carbs you need to eat each day to lose excess weight.

Why would You eat fewer Carbs?

The Dietary Guidelines for Americans recommends that carbs provide 45-65% of the daily calorie consumption for all age ranges and sexes. According to the Food and Drug Administration (FDA), the Daily Value (DV) for carbs is 300 grams each day when eating a 2,000-calorie diet.

Some people reduce their day-by-day carb intake with the purpose of losing weight, reducing to around 50-150 grams each day.

Research shows that low carbohydrate diets could be a part of an effective weight-loss strategy. The dietary plan restricts your intake of carbohydrates - including sugars and starches like bread and pasta - and replaces them with protein, healthy fats, and vegetables.

Studies also show that low carbohydrate diets can reduce a person's appetite, result in them feeding on fewer calories, and help them to lose excess weight easier than in other diets, provided they keep up with the diet. In studies comparing low carbohydrate and zero fat diets, researchers have to actively restrict calories in the reduced fat groups to help make the results comparable, however the low carbohydrate groups remain usually far better. Low carbohydrate diets likewise have benefits that exceed just weight loss. They can help lower blood sugar levels, blood circulation pressure, and triglycerides. They are able to also help raise HDL (good) cholesterol and enhance the pattern of LDL (bad) cholesterol.

Low carbohydrate diets often cause more excess weight loss and improve health in comparison with calorie-restricted, zero fat diets that lots of people still recommend. There's a lot of evidence to aid this notion.

Summary

Many studies show that low carbohydrate diets could be far better and healthier than zero fat diets.

What is a minimal carb diet?

There's no clear definition of what produces a low carbohydrate diet, and what's low for one person may possibly not be low for another.

Carbs intake

A person's optimal carb intake depends upon how old they are, gender, body composition, activity levels, personal preference, food culture, and current metabolic health. People who are physically active and also have more muscle tissue can tolerate far more carbs than people who are sedentary. This particularly pertains to those who execute a large amount of high intensity exercise, like weight lifting or sprinting. Metabolic health can be an essential factor. When people develop metabolic syndrome, obesity, or type 2 diabetes, their carb needs change.

People who get into these categories are less in a position to tolerate a whole lot of carbs.

Summary

The perfect carb intake varies between people, based on activity levels, current metabolic health, and several other factors.

How To Decide Your Daily Carb Intake

If you take away the unhealthiest carb sources from your diet, such as refined wheat and added sugars, you are well on the way to improved health.

However, to unlock the metabolic great things about low carbohydrate diets, additionally you have to restrict additional carb sources. There are no scientific papers that explain how to complement carbohydrate intake to individual needs. The next sections discuss what some dietitians believe about carb intake and fat loss.

Consuming 100-150 Grams each day

That is a moderate carb intake. It could work for those who are lean, active, and trying to remain healthy and keep maintaining their weight. It's possible to lose excess weight as of this - and any - carb intake, nevertheless, you may also have to be conscious of calorie consumption and food portion sizes to lose excess weight.

Carbs you can eat are:

all vegetables, several bits of fruit each day, moderate levels of healthy starches, like potatoes, sweet potatoes, and healthier grains, like rice and oats.

Ingesting 50-100 grams each day

This range could be beneficial if you wish to slim down while keeping some carb sources in the dietary plan. It could also help sustain your weight if you're sensitive to carbs.

Carbs you can eat are:

- a lot of vegetables.,
- 2-3 bits of fruit each day,
- minimal levels of starchy carbs,
- Consuming 20-50 grams each day.

That's where the reduced carb diet has bigger effects on metabolism. That is a possible stove for those who want to lose excess weight fast, or possess metabolic problems, obesity, or diabetes.

Consuming less than 50 grams each day

When eating less than 50 grams each day, your body will get into ketosis, offering energy for the mind via so-called ketone bodies. That is more likely to dampen your appetite and make you shed weight automatically.

Carbs you can eat are:

- plenty of low carbohydrate vegetables,
- some berries, maybe with whipped cream,
- trace carbs from other food stuffs, like avocados, nuts, and seeds.

Remember that a minimal carb diet doesn't mean it's a no-carb diet. There's room for a lot of low carbohydrate vegetables.

It's vital that you experiment

Each individual is exclusive and what works for just one person might not work for another. It's vital that you do some self-experimentation and find out what is most effective for you. When you have type 2 diabetes, speak to your doctor prior to making any adjustments, because the dietary plan can drastically lessen your dependence on medication.

Summary

For those who are physically active or want to keep up their weight, a variety of 100-150 grams of carbs each day may have benefits. For all those aiming to slim down quickly, heading under 50 grams each day under the direction of the doctor may help.

A minimal carb diet isn't only about weight-loss, it could also improve your wellbeing. Because of this, the diet should be based on whole, unprocessed foods and healthy carb sources.

Low Carb Junk Food that are Unhealthy.

If you wish to improve your wellbeing, choose unprocessed foods such as:

- lean meats
- fish
- eggs

- vegetables
- nuts
- avocados
- healthy fats

Choose carbohydrate sources including fiber. If you need a moderate carb consumption, try to select unrefined starch sources, like potatoes, sweet potatoes, oats, and brown rice. Added sugars along with other processed carbs are always unhealthy options, it's recommended that you limit or prevent them.

Summary

It's very vital that you choose healthy, fiber-rich carb sources. A healthy diet plan has a lot of vegetables, even at the cheapest degree of carb intake.

Low Carbohydrate Diets Assist You to Burn Fat

Low carbohydrates diets help reduce your blood degrees of insulin, a hormone that brings the glucose from carbs in to the body's cells.

Among the functions of insulin would be to store up fat. Many experts think that the main reason low carbohydrate diets work so well is that they lessen your degrees of this hormone. One more thing that insulin does would be to tell the kidneys to retain sodium. This is why high carb diets could cause excess fluid retention.

Whenever you cut carbs, you reduce insulin and your kidneys start to shed excess water. It's common for people to lose lots of water weight in the first couple of days on a minimal carb diet. Some dietitians suggest you may lose as much as 5-10 pounds (2.3-4.5 kg) in this manner.

Weight loss will decelerate after the first week, however your fat mass may continue steadily to decrease in the event that you keep up with the diet.

One report compared low carbohydrate and zero fat diets and used DEXA scanners, which have become accurate measures of body composition. The reduced carb dieters lost quite a lot of surplus fat and gained muscle at exactly the same time.

Studies show that low carbohydrate diets are particularly capable of reducing in your abdominal cavity, also called *visceral fat or stomach fat*. This is actually the most dangerous fat and it is strongly connected with many diseases.

If you're not used to low carb diet, you'll probably have to proceed through an adaptation phase where the body is getting used to burning fat rather than carbs. That is called the *"low carbohydrate flu,"* and it's usually over in a few days.

After this initial phase has ended, many people report having more energy than before, without afternoon dips in energy that are normal on high carb diets.

Summary

Water weight drops fast on a minimal carb diet, and weight loss takes a piece longer. It's common to feel sick the first couple of days of cutting your carb intake. However, many people feel good after this initial adaptation phase.

Before starting the reduced carb diet, try tracking how many carbs you take in on an average day and whether they're healthy or unhealthy.

A free app might help. Because fiber doesn't really count number as carbohydrates, you are can exclude the dietary fiber grams from the full total number.

Instead, count net carbs, by using this computation:

Net Carbs = Total Carbs - Fiber.

If you're not slimming down or weight loss slows down throughout the low carbohydrate diet, have a look at these possible explanations why.

Among the advantages of low carbohydrate diets is the fact that, for many people, it's easy to accomplish. You don't have to track anything unless you need to.

Simply eat some protein, healthy fats, and veggies at every meal. Has some nuts, seeds, avocados, and full-fat milk products. Also, choose unprocessed foods.

Fruits and Low-Carb

Most people agree that fruits fit perfectly right into a healthy life-style routine. However, people over a low carb diet have a tendency to prevent fruits. There are even low-carb dieters who head to extremes and say that fruit is downright unhealthy. Meanwhile, most health practitioners and life style professionals advise first timers to eat fruit each day. Because of this, the question whether fruit is acceptable on the low carb diet appears to come up on a regular basis.

The principal goal of low carb diets is carb restriction. This involves restricting the foods which contain probably the most carbohydrates, including candy, sugary carbonated drinks and root vegetables like potatoes, and grain products like pasta and bread. But fruits, regardless of the health halo, also have a tendency to be fairly abundant with carbohydrates, primarily the easy sugars, glucose and fructose.

This is actually the net carb (total carbs - fiber) count for some fruits:

- Grapes (1 cup / 151g) 26 grams
- Banana (1 medium) 24 grams
- Pear (1 medium) 22 grams
- Apple (1 medium) 21 grams
- Pineapple (1 cup / 165g) 20 grams
- Blueberries (1 cup / 148g) 17 grams
- Oranges (1 medium) 12 grams
- Kiwi (1 medium) 9 grams
- Strawberries (1 cup / 144g) 8 grams
- Lemon (1 fruit) 6 grams

Fruits are higher in carbs than low carb veggies but reduced carbs than foods like bread or pasta.

Summary

Fruits are usually saturated in carbs. Because of this, you will need to modest your fruit absorption over a low carb diet.

Pass Your Carb Budget Wisely

It is critical to take into account that not all low carb diets are the same. There is absolutely no obvious definition of just what takes its low carb diet. Whether any person can or will have fruit in their diet depends upon lots of things. This consists of their current goals, activity levels, current metabolic health insurance and personal preference. Someone who aims to eat only 100-150 grams of carbs each day can easily fit into several bits of fruit each day without exceeding their limit.

However, a person who is usually on an extremely low carb ketogenic diet with under 50 grams each day doesn't genuinely have much room.

Rather than spending the complete carb budget on one or two 2 bits of fruit, it might be better spent eating a lot of low carb vegetables that are more nutritious, calorie for calorie.

Summary

Although some fruit intake is okay of all low carb diets, you may want to avoid fruit if you're trying to attain *ketosis*.

How about Fructose?

Fruits taste sweet because they have a combination of *fructose and glucose*. There's been a whole lot of discuss the harmful ramifications of table sugar and high-fructose corn syrup, due to the fact they contain a lot fructose.

Studies also show that excess fructose intake is connected with a variety of health issues, including obesity, type 2 diabetes and metabolic syndrome.

However, the role of fructose continues to be controversial, no strong evidence proves that it's harmful in normal amounts. It's very vital that you recognize that fructose may just end up being harmful in a particular lifestyle context. For those who are inactive and eat a high-carb Western diet, eating a whole lot of fructose could cause harm. But people who are healthy, lean and active are able to eat some fructose. Rather than being converted into fat, it'll go towards replenishing glycogen stores in the liver.

If you are already eating a healthy, real-food based diet with a lot of protein and fat, smaller amounts of fructose from fruit won't cause harm. Fruits also contain fiber, plenty of drinking water and significant chewing resistance. It's extremely difficult to over-eat fructose by just eating fruit. The possible harmful effects of fructose came from added sugars, not from real foods like fruits.

However, juice is a different story. There's without any fiber in it, no chewing resistance and it could contain nearly the same amount of sugar like a soda. Fruit is okay, juice is not.

Summary

Fruit contains an assortment of fructose and glucose. Excessive fructose intake is known as unhealthy, but this simply pertains to added sugar in processed food.

Fruit is Healthy

The ultimate way to enter nutritional ketosis and go through the full metabolic great things about low carb diets is to lessen carbs, usually below 50 grams each day.

This consists of fruit. There are multiple reasons people adopt such a diet plan. Some get it done for health factors such as obesity, diabetes or epilepsy. Others simply feel best eating this way. There is absolutely no reason to discourage these people from avoiding fruit. It doesn't contain any essential nutrients which you can't obtain from vegetables.

Although some low-carbers can do best limiting fruit, exactly the same may not connect with others. Fruits are healthy, unprocessed foods which are abundant with fiber, antioxidants, minerals and vitamins. Fruits are more healthy options compared to the processed foods people are ingesting in their bodies each day.

Summary

Daily intake of fruit is normally recommended in a healthy diet plan. However, for all those carrying out a low carb diet, moderation is key.

Low carb Fruits

Not all fruits are saturated in sugar and carbs. Some are even considered vegetables for their insufficient sweetness. Here are some types of low carb fruits:

- **Tomatoes:** 3.2 g per 100 g (1 tomato).
- **Watermelon:** 7.6 g per 100 g (one-third of the wedge).
- **Strawberries:** 7.7 g per 100 g (two-thirds of any cup).
- **Cantaloupe:** 8.2 g per 100 g (two small wedges).
- **Avocado:** 8.5 g per 100 g (half an avocado).
- **Peaches:** 9.5 g per 100 g (one large peach).

Additionally, berries are often considered acceptable on the low carb diet so long as they may be eaten in moderation.

Summary

Some fruits are relatively lower in carbohydrates and perfectly ideal for people over a low carb diet. Had in these are tomatoes, watermelon, avocado and different berries. People on low carb or ketogenic diets may choose to avoid most fruit, as it could prevent ketosis. Several low carb exceptions have avocados, tomatoes plus some berries.

For all those not carrying out a low carb diet, fruits are well balanced meals that can make a healthy, real-food based diet.

Chapter 11

Low Carb Kitchen Gadgets

The best low carb kitchen gadgets you should have to be successful on the diet and which will make life easier. This list might seem daunting, but once you've these essentials in your kitchen, they'll make your daily life so easier. Whether it's food prepping, baking, or making a delicious low carb meal, these kitchen gadgets can help make the procedure seamless and fun!

Silicone Bakeware

Using silicone moulds over traditional tin bakeware has sort of changed my entire life. Low carb cooked goods are usually just a little fragile, particularly when warm. It is because nut flours such as almond or coconut flour lack gluten. Silicone moulds are flexible and you'll have no problem releasing bread or muffins. Forget about paper cups either!

Kitchen Scales

So handy for measuring ingredients. Kitchen scales takes all of the guesswork out of cooking and baking. For a few recipes, it's essential that you adhere to the right amount of ingredients.

Measuring Cups and Measuring Spoons

Another best option to kitchen scales. In the United Kingdom ingredients are usually measured in grams and litres, however in the United States cups are trusted. You will find zillions of awesome low carbohydrate and Keto recipes online. Several are by US based bloggers, so even though you're in the United Kingdom, get hold of a group of US cups which means you won't miss out! And if you believe spoons - how many different sizes of teaspoons and tablespoons do you have in drawer? Those are for eating, not for cooking.

Spiralizer

You never thought I'd say this, but a spiralizer is really a seriously useful gadget. You can spiralize all sorts of vegetables into noodles, from *courgettes to kohlrabi*. No, it won't make zucchini taste the same as spaghetti - but it'll transform them right into a delicious and far healthier alternative. If you put in a sauce such as my low carbohydrate Bolognese sauce, you might have an awesome your meal.

Non-stick Frying Pan

In a minimal carb kitchen, we're not afraid of frying stuff - fat is our friend! You might have tried expensive stainless frying pans (made everything stick) and cheap coated supermarket pans which got scratched immediately. Finally, I went and bought a good nonstick frying pan, which has been my best friend since. I use it for a lot of dishes, from low carbohydrate crepes to the chicken green curry recipe. As well as for eggs - just about any day.

Stick Blender

Hand immersion blenders are simple to use and don't have up much space. I'd say they are the minimum blending equipment in a minimal carb kitchen and also have to admit, I have mine even on holidays. Sometimes, a fork will not do!

Glass Storage Containers

Eating low carbohydrate offers made me are more organized with regards to meal prep. Nipping out to the supermarket to get a ready meal or ordering in a takeaway isn't a choice. Instead, I'm now making double and triple portions of everything and sticking the surplus in the freezer. I want to use less plastic and use glass containers for storage instead.

Food Processor

Amazing to make dough, cauliflower rice, slicing and shredding vegetables. Forget about teary eyes from chopping onions! Spend money on one. It doesn't need to cost the planet earth.

Figure Out How to Enjoy Your Slow Cooker

If you know you'll be home late but have some time in the morning (and even the night time before), use your slow cooker. Slow cookers are a fabulous way to transform cheaper cuts of meat into satisfying comfort meals. That is easy 'set and forget' cooking.

Baking Mat

If you wish to upgrade from baking/parchment paper, a baking mat is invaluable. You may make low carbohydrate pizza onto it, breads or cookies - nothing, nothing, nothing will ever stick. Choose good quality, they are really worth it.

Power Blender

When you can afford to get several £££, you should buy a power blender for your low carbohydrate kitchen. I've got the Optimum Vac2 Vacuum Blender by Froothie. It's a beast. It creates nut butter and soup effortlessly and it produces the smoothest of smoothies. The thing which makes this blender stick out is its vacuum function. Before blending it sucks all air from the container and prevents fruit and veggies from oxidizing. This implies all nutrients are intact, there's no layer separation as well as your smoothies don't change color after a short while.

Ways To Stay Low on Carbohydrate When You Don't Want to Cook

How will you stay low on carbohydrate or keto when you don't want to cook? What now? When you get back late, tired, or you're simply unprepared?

Below are the best ideas for how to stay low on carbohydrate if you don't feel like cooking or don't have time to cook.

Drink coffee or tea

A soothing cup of coffee or tea may be sufficient to limit your appetite, particularly if you then add heavy cream or melted butter. This might take you to the next planned meal, without cooking.

Eat low carb snacks

Fill your pantry and fridge with low carb essentials and that means you can quickly produce a platter with a number of the low carb snacks rather than cooking. Make sure to have at least one protein source.

- Canned fish (tuna, salmon, sardines).
- Selection of cheeses.
- Deli meat or cold cuts 2.
- Avocado.

- Nuts (Which are the best? Have a look at our guide.).
- Frozen berries or other low carb fruits.
- Cream.
- Pate.
- Beef jerky or pork rinds (without sugars or wheat).
- Full-fat yoghurt.
- Olives.
- Mayonnaise.
- Healthy fats - like olive oil - to drizzle over snacks such as mozzarella or veggies.

Reheat leftovers

Get the habit of making double as well as triple meals and vegetables. Freeze the leftovers. Meals are waiting, prepared to reheat, after you don't desire to cook. Leftovers are great for lunches too.

Do minimal cooking

Boil an egg. Fry a steak or buy a hot cooked chicken (without bread stuffing or sweet sauces). Put in a bag of salad, an array of cheeses and homemade mayonnaise.

Supper could be ready in ten minutes. Be creative with salads and use your low carb pantry essentials.

Fast intermittently

Are you truly hungry? Figure out how to satisfy your appetite and eat only when hungry. It is not a choice for a family group but is ideal for people. And there is absolutely no faster (pun intended) or simpler option.

Note

Get the second book in the series for access to all the flavorful recipes.

Low Carb Diet: 100 Essential Flavorful Recipes For Quick & Easy Low-Carb Homemade Cooking

Free Bonus

Download my **"Keto Cookbook with 60+ Keto Recipes For Your Personal Enjoyment"** Ebook For **FREE!**

The **Keto Diet Cookbook** is a collection of **60+ delicious recipes** that are easy and fun to make in the comfort of your own home. It gives you the exact *recipes that you can use to prepare meals for any moment of the day, breakfast, lunch, dinner, and even dessert.*

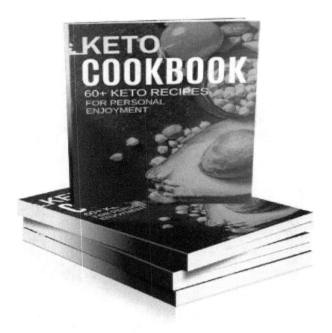

You don't need 5 different cookbooks with a ton of recipes to live a healthy and fun lifestyle. *You just need a*

good and efficient one and that is what the **Keto Diet Cookbook** *is.*

Click the URL below to Download the Book For FREE, and also Subscribe for Free books, giveaways, and new releases by me. https://mayobook.com/drmichelle

Feedback

I'd like to express my gratitude to you for choosing to read this book, Thank you. I hope you got what you wanted from it. Your feedback as to whether I succeeded or not is greatly appreciated, as I went to great lengths to make it as helpful as possible.

I would be grateful if you could write me a review on the product detail page about how this book has helped you. Your review means a lot to me, as I would love to hear about your successes. Nothing makes me happier than knowing that my work has aided someone in achieving their goals and progressing in life; which would likewise motivate me to improve and serve you better, and also encourage other readers to get influenced positively by my work. Your feedback means so much to me, and I will never take it for granted.

However, if there is something you would love to tell me as to improve on my work, it is possible that you are not impressed enough, or you have a suggestion, errors, recommendation, or criticism for us to improve on; we are profoundly sorry for your experience (remember, we are human, we are not perfect, and we are constantly striving to improve).

Rather than leaving your displeasure feedback on the retail product page of this book, please send your feedback, suggestion, or complaint to us via E-mail to **"michelle@mayobook.com"** so that action can be taken quickly to ensure necessary correction, improvement, and implementation for the better reading experience.

I'm honored that you've read this book and that you enjoy it. I strive to provide you with the best reading experience possible.

Thank you, have a wonderful day!

About The Author

I help people to eat healthy food and live healthier lives. I have been a registered dietitian since 2005. In the past decade, I have helped hundreds of people to improve their health and wellbeing through nutrition. I am a licensed dietitian in the state of California and a member of the American Dietetic Association. I have been working in the wellness industry for over 10 years, and I have worked with people who have type 2 diabetes, high blood pressure, heart disease, weight gain, metabolic syndrome, and cancer. I understand that nutrition is key to good health, and I love helping people eat well.

My goal is to help people get healthy by providing them with a balanced diet, lifestyle changes, and support. My approach is holistic, which means that I look at diet as a whole, rather than focusing on one aspect.

I am a holistic nutritionist. I help people change their eating habits and lifestyles so they can achieve and maintain a healthy weight and a happy, energetic lifestyle. I teach people how to eat well, and I help people find the balance between healthy food and food that they love. I also work with people who have cancer, diabetes, and other chronic conditions to help them live healthier lives. I offer personalized nutrition counseling and healthy meal planning. I have a master's degree in nutrition and a doctorate in nutritional science. I am a registered dietitian in the state of California and a member of the American Dietetic Association. I believe in a healthy lifestyle, and I help people find the best path to get there.

Subscribe to my Newsletter to download my Free Book, and also be informed about my new releases, and giveaways here: https://mayobook.com/drmichelle

Connect with me on my Facebook Page here: https://fb.me/MichelleEllenGleen

Other Books

1. Low Carb Diet: 100 Essential Flavorful Recipes For Quick & Easy Low-Carb Homemade Cooking
2. Low Carb Diet: A Complete Guide to a Healthy Lifestyle Using Real Foods and Real Science, How it Works, How to Start, & More!
3. Alkaline Diet: The Secret to Healthy Living with Alkaline Foods (Healthy Food Lifestyle)
4. Brain Cancer Awareness: How to Help Your Brain Fight Brain Cancer
5. Trigger Points: The New Self Treatment Guide to Pain Relief
6. Skin Tag Removal: How To Get Rid of Your Skin Tags in Simple Steps
7. Apple Cider Vinegar: A Quick, Easy, and Affordable Guide to the Health Benefits, and Healing Power of Apple Cider Vinegar (ACV)
8. Apple Cider Vinegar: The Amazing Guide on The Uses of ACV For Numerous Health Conditions, and How to Make it from Home
9. Dr. Sebi Cookbook: Alkaline Diet Nutritional Guide with Sea moss, Medicinal Herbal Teas, Smoothies, Desserts, Mushroom, Salads, Soups & More, to ... with 100+ Recipes

10. The Alkaline Diet Cookbook: Your Guide to Eating More Alkaline Foods, and Less Acidic Foods For Healthy Living (Healthy Food Lifestyle)

11. Ketogenic Diet For Beginners: Your Complete Keto Guide and Cookbook with Low Carb, High-Fat Recipes For Living The Keto Lifestyle

12. Anti Inflammatory Diet Cookbook For Beginners: 3-Week Quick & Delicious Meal Plan with Easy Recipes to Heal The Immune Systems and Restore Overall Health

CPSIA information can be obtained
at www.ICGtesting.com
Printed in the USA
BVHW031013061022
648827BV00013B/156